MENOPAUSE

WEIGHT LOSS AND

BEYOND

Your Quick Start Guide to Losing Weight Gaining
Strength and Embracing Change

MICHELLE A BATES

DEDICATION

To my husband John, my rock, my heart, my everything. Thank you for not letting menopause scare you away. This book wouldn't exist without your patience, love, and unwavering support. Thank you for your encouragement and for being my partner in every sense of the word. You are such a beautiful soul, and I am grateful that God brought you into my life. You inspire me every day. Don't ever stop.

To my mom, whose strength and love have shaped me into the woman I am today. Your resilience and kindness to others are a source of endless inspiration. I love you deeply.

To the women who shared their stories and struggles, inspiring me to write this book. Your courage is my motivation.

This book is for all of us who are still learning, adapting, and growing and refuse to be defined by age or limitations. Together, we can turn this chapter into our best yet.

A NOTE FROM THE AUTHOR

Hello Beautiful! I am so glad you're here, holding this book in your hands because it means you're ready to take control of your journey through menopause. I know firsthand how challenging and even overwhelming this time can feel. Maybe you're dealing with weight gain that seems unmovable, or maybe your emotions are shifting in ways you didn't expect. Perhaps, like many of us, you're simply feeling at odds with the body you thought you knew. I understand deeply because I've been right where you are, and I wrote this book to share everything I've learned along the way—along with the insights of countless women I've had the privilege to work with.

One of the most common and frustrating changes during menopause is weight gain. And this isn't just about appearance—it's about feeling comfortable, capable, and in control. As our bodies change, so do the "rules" we've always followed for weight loss, fitness, and wellness. This book is here to help you navigate those changes with clarity, to support your physical health and emotional resilience, and to guide you toward a place where you feel at ease and empowered in your own skin.

Menopause can present unexpected hurdles: stubborn weight, emotional shifts that seem out of the blue, and physical changes that might feel bewildering. I designed this book as a straightforward, supportive guide—something simple and heartfelt that addresses what matters most to us during this time. I know you don't have time to wade through an overwhelming amount of information. Instead, we'll focus on practical tools, helpful insights, and the essentials that make the biggest difference.

In the chapters ahead, we'll look at the many layers of menopause—physical, emotional, and mental. You'll find information to help you understand what's happening in your body and, even more importantly, how to respond in a way that feels empowering and manageable. This isn't an end; it's the start of a new chapter filled with potential, strength, and resilience.

I've included a 10-Day Rapid Weight Loss Plan, designed to help you see results quickly and to show you the power of small, consistent changes. For many, this initial progress can be one of the most motivating aspects of their journey. If upon completing the book, you're wanting to go even deeper, my Menopause Weight Loss Blueprint offers a complete, step-by-step program that provides structure for long-term health and lasting change. I mention it here as an option because I want you to have the tools you need, whether you're looking for just a bit of guidance or a full support system. You're in control.

The truth is, menopause isn't the same for everyone, and this book is here to honor that. You may be feeling frustrated with weight gain, overwhelmed by hot flashes, or struggling with low energy and motivation. My hope is that as you read, reflect, and engage with these tools, you'll feel seen, understood, and fully supported. I want this to feel like a personal conversation between us, one woman to another, letting you know you're not alone in this. Together, we'll embrace this stage of life not as something to dread but as a time to become our strongest, healthiest, most empowered selves.

Thank you for allowing me to be a part of your journey. Take a deep breath, and let's begin.

TABLE OF CONTENTS

CHAPTER 1

A Journey Long Overdue

"
"The beginning is the most important part of the work." — **Plato**
"

D id you know that over 1 billion women are expected to experience menopause by 2025? Yet, for so many, this natural stage of life remains shrouded in misunderstanding and silence.

For generations, menopause has been treated as a "condition" rather than a transition. It's often something we're expected to endure quietly, as though it's a personal failure rather than a natural part of aging. Society has conditioned us to see it as the beginning of decline rather than the start of a powerful new chapter.

My own journey into understanding menopause began much the same way. The first time I ever thought about it seriously was when I saw Clair Huxtable, an icon of strength and elegance, dealing with it on an episode of The Cosby Show. I was young, and menopause felt far off—something that happened to "older" women. To me, it was just one of those mysterious things that happened as people got older, something almost comical. I remember Clair putting her head in the freezer to cool off, laughing along with the laugh track, but what I didn't realize then was that the show was shedding light on something that would become very real for me one day.

I didn't think about menopause again for a long time. I was focused on life, career, family, and helping my clients reach their weight loss goals. But then something changed. One day, I found myself struggling with my own weight in a way I hadn't before. The techniques I'd always relied on weren't working anymore. My clients were struggling too, and I could sense their frustration. They would come to me saying, "I'm doing everything right, but the scale isn't moving." For some reason, it felt like we were all fighting an invisible battle.

It wasn't until I went to see a weight loss doctor myself that the reality of what was happening hit me. After my blood tests came back, the doctor told me, "You're premenopausal. Your hormone levels are changing, and it's going to affect your weight, your energy, your sleep—pretty much everything." I was blindsided. No one had ever mentioned to me that this was coming, that this was something I should prepare for. I'd gone in hoping for a quick answer to why I wasn't losing weight like before, and I left with a new, unexpected chapter unfolding before me.

In that moment, I realized I wasn't just dealing with a personal struggle—I was facing the same thing that millions of women would go through. I knew right then that I needed to dig deeper, not just for myself but for the clients who trusted me to guide them. My role as a coach was suddenly much bigger. I wasn't just helping women lose weight; I was now on a mission to help women understand the profound changes their bodies would go through and to provide real answers that they weren't getting elsewhere.

As I started researching, I was stunned by how little information and support there was. The options felt bleak: take hormones, face scary risks, or try to "manage" with antidepressants and medications that seemed like a band-aid rather than a solution. The more I looked, the more frustrated I became. Why wasn't anyone talking about lifestyle changes, dietary shifts, or holistic approaches? Why weren't we being taught how to manage menopause naturally, in a way that empowered us?

A Culture of Silence

It quickly became clear to me that menopause was a taboo topic. Talking about menopause was often met with discomfort, and there was a sense that it was something to hide. I found this silence frustrating and, frankly, damaging. By keeping menopause in the shadows, we weren't just ignoring a biological reality—we were undermining women's well-being.

Historically, women in menopause were often viewed as "less than." Society painted a picture of menopause as a time when women became invisible, irrelevant, or even hysterical. There was a time when women were even institutionalized or dismissed as "unwell" simply for showing the symptoms of menopause. Can you imagine that? Instead of receiving support and understanding, they were treated as though they were mentally unstable. And while we've come a long way since then, the shadow of that stigma still lingers.

This realization lit a fire in me. Too many women were going through this and going through it alone and with the wrong idea. I wanted to help women see menopause for what it truly is: a powerful time of self-discovery, resilience, and strength. This wasn't about enduring menopause; it was about thriving and properly navigating through it, about reclaiming our health and redefining what it means to age and do so ever so gracefully.

The Road to Reclaiming Control

One of the most important lessons I learned was that menopause doesn't have to mean losing control. Yes, our bodies change. Yes, things get harder. But with the right tools, knowledge, and support, we can adapt. We can take control of our health, navigate these changes gracefully, and come out the other side stronger than ever.

This is what I wanted to offer women: the confidence and the tools to reclaim their bodies and peace of mind. Through research, I began to piece together an approach that combined nutrition, exercise, mindset, and lifestyle changes tailored specifically for the menopausal body. I started testing this approach with clients, refining it with each step, and the results spoke for themselves. Women were feeling better, seeing the changes in their bodies, and embracing this stage of life with a renewed sense of beauty, strength, and wisdom.

What You'll Find in This Book

This book is my answer to the silence, the stigma, and the lack of support that so many women experience during menopause. I'm here to tell you that you're not alone, you're not going crazy, and there is a way to feel good again. In these pages, I've created a clear path forward—a path that doesn't just focus on surviving menopause, but on thriving through it.

Throughout these chapters, I'm going to take you through the key elements of managing menopause:

- Understanding the Stages of Menopause: Knowledge is empowering. We'll explore perimenopause, menopause, and post-menopause, so you'll know exactly what's happening in your body and what to expect.
- Nutrition Strategies Tailored for Menopause: We'll discuss how to nourish your body in ways that support your hormonal balance, boost your metabolism, and promote weight loss.
- Exercise and Strength Training: Movement is medicine, and we'll go through how strength training and other exercises can transform your body and mind, no matter what age or stage of menopause you're in.

- Stress and Sleep Management: I'll guide you through tools and techniques to improve your quality of sleep and reduce stress, which play a critical role in overall health and well-being.
- Mindset and Self-Care: This journey is as much about mental resilience as it is about physical health. Together, we'll work on building a mindset that embraces change with grace and positivity.

You'll find real, actionable steps that will empower you to reclaim your health and redefine your experience of menopause. I'm here to guide you, every step of the way, as you take control of this journey.

Key Points

- Menopause as a New Beginning: Menopause isn't an end but rather a new chapter in life, filled with opportunities for growth, transformation, and self-care.
- Redefining the Narrative: Shifting the perspective on menopause helps break down cultural stigmas, allowing women to approach this stage with positivity and strength.
- Empowerment through Knowledge: Understanding menopause empowers women to take control of their health, happiness, and self-confidence during this phase.
- Celebrating Change: Embracing the physical and emotional changes of menopause can lead to a deeper appreciation for the wisdom and resilience that come with age.
- Setting the Stage for a Positive Journey: This chapter encourages a mindset shift, helping women look forward to the journey ahead with optimism and a focus on well-being.

Reflection & Personal Insights

Take a moment to reflect on how this chapter resonates with your own experiences. Use the prompts below to guide your thoughts, and feel free to jot down any other reflections that come to mind.

1. How do I currently feel about entering (or being in) menopause?

- (Write about any emotions, beliefs, or expectations you have about this new stage of life. Do you see it as a beginning or an end?)

_____

_____

_____

_____

_____

2. What positive changes would I like to focus on as I move forward?

- (Identify one or two areas of your life where you want to make positive shifts, whether it's physical health, emotional well-being, or something else entirely.)

_____

_____

_____

_____

_____

3. What myths or fears do I need to let go of?

- (Consider any cultural beliefs or misconceptions about menopause that may be holding you back. Write down anything you're ready to release.)

---

4. Affirmation for this Chapter:

- (Create a short, positive affirmation that speaks to how you want to approach menopause. For example: "I embrace this new beginning with strength and gratitude.")

Use the space on the next page to capture your thoughts, reflections, or anything else that came up for you in this chapter.

Notes

CHAPTER 2

Understanding the Three Stages of Menopause

"Life is a series of natural and spontaneous changes.
Don't resist them; that only creates sorrow.
Let reality be reality." — **Lao Tzu**

So, being honest, when it comes to menopause—most of us didn't really understand what it was all about until we were right in the middle of it. I mean really, how many of us grew up actually knowing the details? I must admit, for years I thought menopause was just a stage of a woman's life that happened way off in the future. You'd have a few hot flashes, your period would stop, and then life would go back to normal, right? Wrong.

There's so much more to menopause than that, and here's the clincher—it isn't just one isolated event. Menopause is a transition that unfolds in three distinct stages: perimenopause, menopause, and post-menopause. Each stage of menopause brings its own set of changes, challenges, and lessons to be learned and endured.

Here's something that might surprise you and most certainly surprised me, once you hit menopause, you're in it for the rest of your life. That's right, menopause is a permanent shift, not just a passing phase. When I first realized that, it stopped me in my tracks. I thought, Why didn't I know this? Why didn't anyone tell me this sooner? *And furthermore, why isn't this being taken more seriously?*

The truth is, so many of us enter this phase feeling blindsided and somewhat betrayed by our bodies. We wonder, *What's happening to my body? Why doesn't anyone talk about this in more detail?* I hear it all the time from the women I've coached, and honestly, I have to admit, I've been there too.

That's why understanding the three stages of menopause is so important. Knowledge is power. When you understand what's happening to your body, you can take control instead of feeling like your body is controlling you. So let's dive in.

Perimenopause: The Beginning of the Shift

Let's start with perimenopause, the first stage of "The change". This is where all the changes begin, and for some of us, it feels like being caught off guard. Perimenopause can sneak up on you as early as your mid-30s, but for most women, it begins in their 40s.

What's happening? Your hormones, especially estrogen and progesterone are starting to fluctuate. These may be subtle changes at first, or they may hit you like a ton of bricks.

Perimenopause can last anywhere from a few months to over a decade. Yes, that's right, a decade.

Here's the thing, every woman's experience is different. Some women sail through it with hardly any symptoms at all, while others feel like their entire world has been flipped upside down.

Signs of Perimenopause

- **Irregular periods**: Your cycles may become unpredictable, shorter, longer, heavier, or lighter. Take your pick, I personally experienced it all.
- **Hot flashes and night sweats**: These sudden waves of heat can leave you drenched in sweat and wondering what's going on. I can't tell you how many times I asked my husband "Babe are you hot too?"
- **Mood swings**: You might find yourself laughing one minute and crying the next, with no clear reason. Again, girl yes, that is totally normal, and no, you are not crazy!
- **Sleep disruptions**: Insomnia or waking up multiple times a night can also become a regular struggle.
- **Weight gain and body changes**: You might notice weight creeping up, especially around your midsection.

These symptoms are your body's way of signaling that change is happening. And while it can feel overwhelming, knowing what's behind these changes can help you navigate them with more confidence and less fear. You see, knowledge is power!

Menopause: The Milestone Moment

Menopause is the big milestone—12 consecutive months without a period. This officially marks the end of your reproductive years. For most women, menopause happens around age 51, but keep in mind, it can occur earlier or later. Our bodies are all different so how menopause affects each one of us will be different.

By this point, your ovaries have stopped releasing eggs, and your body is producing much lower levels of estrogen and progesterone. While menopause itself is a moment in time, the symptoms leading up to and following it can linger.

What Menopause May Bring

- **Ongoing symptoms**: Hot flashes, mood swings, and sleep disruptions may still be part of your life.
- **Physical changes**: Hormonal shifts can bring changes in your skin, energy levels, and overall health.
- **Body Shape:** You may also notice that as your midsection is increasing in size, you are decreasing in size from the waist down, particularly your bum and your legs. Yep, that's normal too, but do not despair, there are thing we can do to counter that (we'll discuss that in an upcoming chapter)

For some women, menopause feels like a relief—no more periods, no more uncertainty. For others, it's a bittersweet transition. You might grieve the end of a chapter, or you might feel liberated. However you feel is valid.

Post-Menopause: The New Normal

Once you've crossed that 12-month milestone, you're officially in postmenopause, and this stage lasts for the rest of your life. Yes, you are in postmenopause for the rest of your life. While your hormone levels may have stabilized, the effects of lower estrogen can increase your risk for certain conditions, like osteoporosis and heart disease.

But postmenopause isn't all about risks—it's also a time of newfound stability and strength. Many women find this stage brings a renewed sense of confidence, clarity and freedom from the monthly visitor.

Taking Care of Yourself in Postmenopause

- **Focus on long-term health**: Prioritize nutrition, exercise, mental health and lifestyle choices to support your body and mind.
- **Health screenings**: Stay on top of regular check-ups to keep your bones, heart, and overall health in check.
- **Support your cognitive health:** I can not stress how important it is to stay active, challenge your brain regularly with puzzles, social interaction and by learning new skills. Feed your brain with a nutrient rich diet and supplementation when necessary (like taking 1000 mg of Omega-3s a day) and prioritize getting 8 hours of sleep to help maintain a healthy weight and mental sharpness.

This stage is all about creating a healthy, vibrant future for yourself. You've earned the wisdom and resilience that come with experience, and now it's time to put that all to work and start truly enjoying it

Why Understanding These Stages Matters

Like we discussed earlier, when you understand the stages of menopause, you can stop feeling blindsided or overwhelmed. Instead, you can approach each phase with clarity, confidence, and a solid plan. Knowledge puts you back in the driver's seat so burn rubber!

Common Myths About Menopause

- **Myth #1**: Menopause happens overnight. *Reality*: It's a gradual process that happens over the course of many years.
- **Myth #2**: Weight gain is inevitable and permanent. *Reality*: Inevitable, almost always yes, but permanent absolutely not. With the right lifestyle changes, you can not only lose menopausal weight, but manage it.
- **Myth #3**: Menopause only affects physical health. *Reality*: Emotional and mental health are deeply affected by this transition.
- **Myth #4**: HRT is the only solution. *Reality*: If your choice is to avoid HRT, there are many ways to navigate menopause, from lifestyle changes to alternative treatments.

Menopause doesn't have to be a scary or isolating experience. With the right information and support, it can be a time of great strength and incredible growth, empowerment, and transformation.

Reflection & Personal Insights

Now it's time to reflect on how this chapter's insights apply to your own experiences. Use the prompts below to help guide your thoughts.

1. What stage of menopause do I feel I'm in right now based on what I've read?

(Reflect on how this understanding shifts your perspective on what you're currently experiencing.)

_____

_____

_____

_____

2. Which myths about menopause have I believed or encountered?

(Think about any misconceptions that may have shaped your view of menopause and how challenging these beliefs could change your perspective.)

_____

_____

_____

_____

3. What fears or concerns do I have about this journey?

(Consider any fears related to menopause, and think about how reframing these could make a difference in your journey.)

_____

_____

_____

_____

_____

_____

4. How have weight gain and body changes affected me personally?

(Reflect on how physical changes have impacted your emotions, confidence, or lifestyle. No PC answers, dig deep and answer with complete honesty)

_____

_____

_____

_____

_____

_____

5. What actions can I take to strengthen my mental and emotional resilience?

(Identify one or two ways to nurture your mental and emotional well-being as you navigate menopause.)

_____

_____

_____

_____

_____

_____

_____

_____

_____

_____

_____

NOTES:

Use the space on the next page to capture your thoughts, reflections, or anything else that came up for you in this chapter.

Notes

CHAPTER 3

Navigating the Symptoms of Menopause with Confidence

"You don't have to control your thoughts. You just have to stop letting them control you"

— Dan Millman

et's talk about the elephant in the room: symptoms. When we think of menopause, the first things that come to mind are hot flashes, mood swings, and sleepless nights. It's the stuff of legends, right? The things we've heard about but maybe didn't really understand until they started happening to us. And for some of us, it's been one of those "Oh, this is what they were talking about!" moments.

But here's the thing: yes, menopause has symptoms, and yes, they can be frustrating, uncomfortable, even downright annoying. But they don't have to control your life. In fact, with the right tools and a bit of understanding, you can navigate these changes with confidence. You don't have to suffer in silence, and you don't have to feel like your body is working against you. Because, honestly? Your body is just adapting, adjusting to a new way of being.

In this chapter, we're going to break down some of the most common menopause symptoms and look at ways to manage them that are practical, doable, and don't require a complete life overhaul. We're talking about real, sustainable changes that can help you feel more like yourself again. Because menopause doesn't get to define us—we define how we move through it.

Hot Flashes and Night Sweats: Tackling the Heat

Let's start with the classic symptom: hot flashes. These aren't just a little warmth—they can feel like you've got an internal furnace that someone cranked up to high without warning. And when they hit at night, leading to night sweats, it can leave you feeling like you've just run a marathon in your pajamas.

One thing to remember is that hot flashes and night sweats are all about the body's thermostat being a bit off-kilter. Your hormones, especially estrogen, help regulate your body temperature. So when estrogen levels dip, it can throw that temperature regulation out the window.

Here are a few strategies that might help:

- Layer up: Dressing in layers allows you to peel off a layer when you feel a flash coming on. As you remove layers, you're allowing your body to cool down faster, and since cold chills often follow hot flashes, it's easier to put the layers back on to stay comfortable.

- Stay cool: Keep a small fan on your bedside table, or even better, a handheld fan you can carry with you during the day.
- Avoid triggers: Spicy foods, caffeine, alcohol, and stress are common culprits for hot flashes. I'm not saying you can't enjoy these things, but just be mindful of when and how much you're consuming.
- Mindfulness and deep breathing: Studies have shown that deep breathing exercises can reduce the frequency and intensity of hot flashes. So when you feel one coming on, try taking a few slow, deep breaths.

Hot flashes don't have to own you. These tips won't necessarily eliminate them entirely, but they can help you feel more in control when they happen.

Mood Swings and Emotional Changes: Finding Balance

Next up is the emotional roller coaster. One minute you're fine, and the next, you're tearing up at a commercial or snapping at your partner because they didn't put their socks in the laundry.

Mood swings are real, and they're exhausting.

Hormonal shifts impact our neurotransmitters—those little chemical messengers in our brain. So when estrogen and progesterone levels are all over the place, it can affect our mood, and sometimes quite drastically.

What can you do to help find a bit more emotional balance?

- Exercise: Moving your body by performing some sort of exercise releases endorphins, which can help boost your mood. And you don't have to do anything extreme, even a walk around the block or a bit of stretching can make a huge difference.
- Mindful moments: Take time each day to do something that calms you, whether it's meditating, journaling, or just sitting quietly reading a book with a cup of tea.
- Stay connected: Talking to friends or loved ones about what you're experiencing can be a huge relief. Sometimes just knowing you're not alone is enough to make the tough moments feel a little less heavy.
- Consider taking natural supplements: Some women find relief with supplements like magnesium (200–400 mg daily), vitamin B6 (50–100 mg daily), or herbal options like St. John's Wort or black cohosh. But remember to check with your healthcare provider before starting anything new.

Mood swings can make you feel like you're out of control, but with a few intentional changes, you can bring a bit more calm and stability back into your days.

Sleep Disruptions: Prioritizing Rest

Ah, sleep. Remember when you used to go to bed and wake up feeling rested? For many women in menopause, those days feel like a very distant memory. Insomnia, waking up multiple times a night, or just not getting good-quality sleep are common symptoms that can leave you feeling drained.

Lack of sleep doesn't just make you tired; it can affect everything from your mood to cognitive function to your weight. So, making sleep a priority is one of the best things you can do for your overall well-being.

Here are some tips for getting better sleep during menopause:

- Create a bedtime routine: Just like you'd create a wind-down routine for a child, give yourself that same care. Set a regular bedtime, start using blue blocker glasses at night time when watching tv, using your cell phone or computer. Turn off all screens at least an hour before bed, and find relaxing activities like reading or taking a warm bath with epsom salt before bed.
- Keep it cool: A cooler room can make a big difference, especially if you're dealing with night sweats. Lower the thermostat, use breathable bedding, and maybe even sleep with a fan on. This also helps improve your metabolism so it's a win, win.
- Limit caffeine and alcohol: Both can mess with your sleep quality, especially if you have them later in the day.
- Try natural sleep aids: For sleep support, consider melatonin (3-5 mg about 30-60 minutes before bed), GABA (750 mg 30-60 minutes before bed), and 5-HTP (200 mg
- 30-60 minutes before bed) to help with relaxation and better sleep quality. As always, check with a healthcare provider before starting any new supplements.

Making small adjustments to your sleep environment and habits can make a significant difference in how rested you feel each day.

Weight Gain: Navigating the Scale

Now, let's talk about something that comes up in nearly every conversation I have with clients: weight gain. Menopause seems to invite extra pounds, particularly around the midsection, and it's not just about appearances. Carrying extra weight can negatively impact your health, energy levels, and even your confidence.

The good news? While weight gain during menopause can be common, and even inevitable, it does not have to be permanent. You can take control of your body and set yourself up for success.

Here are some starting points:

- Focus on protein: Protein helps keep you full and supports muscle maintenance, which is especially important as we age.
- Incorporate strength training: Building muscle through resistance exercises can help boost your metabolism and keep your bones strong. There is no way around this ladies, so make it a "must do" not a maybe.
- Stay active: Find ways to move every day, whether it's a walk, yoga, or a quick workout. Consistency is key. Can I get an amen?
- Mindful eating: Pay attention to hunger and fullness cues, and try to avoid mindless snacking. Eating with intention can make a big difference.

Weight management during menopause is possible, and it's all about finding a balance that feels sustainable for you.

Brain Fog: Staying Sharp

Lastly, let's touch on brain fog—the frustrating forgetfulness, the mental blanks that make you feel like you're losing your edge. Brain fog can make it hard to focus, remember things, or stay organized, and it's a symptom that often catches women off guard.

While it's frustrating, brain fog isn't permanent, and there are ways to keep your mind sharp:

- Stay active: Physical activity doesn't just benefit the body; it benefits the brain too. Exercise boosts blood flow to the brain and supports cognitive function.
- Challenge your mind: Keep your brain engaged with activities that make you think, like puzzles, reading, or learning something new.
- Prioritize sleep: Lack of sleep can make brain fog worse, so make rest a priority.
- Eat for brain health: Foods rich in omega-3s, like salmon once a week and walnuts, and antioxidant-rich fruits and veggies can support cognitive health.

Remember, brain fog is a normal part of the menopause journey for many women, but it's not something you just have to accept. Remember, small changes can make a big difference.

Empowering Yourself Through Knowledge

At the end of the day, understanding these symptoms is about more than just learning how to "fix" things. It's about taking control of your menopause journey and not letting these changes define who you are. Yes, there will be challenges, but you have the power to navigate them with confidence, clarity, and grace.

Each symptom we face in menopause is a signal from our body, a reminder that we're going through a powerful transformation. And just like any other stage of life, there are ways to handle it, to adapt, and to thrive. This chapter is your reminder that you are stronger than any symptom, and you have all the tools within you to make this time as positive as possible.

In the next chapter, we'll take a deeper dive into how nutrition and hormonal health can become powerful allies in your menopause journey. Together, we'll explore how nourishing your body with the right foods, balancing your macronutrients, and making small, intentional changes can support your hormonal health, boost your energy, and help you feel empowered. This next step is all about discovering how food can work with your body, not against it. You've got this!

Key Points

1. Understanding and Embracing Change: Menopause symptoms, from hot flashes to mood swings, are a natural part of this life stage. Recognizing them as signals from your body can help you approach them with curiosity and self-compassion rather than frustration.

2. Practical Strategies for Symptom Management: From cooling techniques for hot flashes to exercises that support mental and physical well-being, small adjustments can have a big impact on how you experience menopause symptoms day-to-day.

3. The Role of Supplements: Certain supplements, such as magnesium for relaxation or melatonin for sleep, can support symptom relief and overall well-being. Understanding how these can fit into your lifestyle can help you feel more empowered in managing menopause.

4. Mindfulness in the Moment: Tools like mindful breathing, journaling, and setting boundaries can help create a sense of control and peace, especially during emotional ups and downs.

5. The Power of Rest and Recovery: Prioritizing quality sleep and stress management practices is essential for balancing mood, energy, and overall health during menopause. These habits can form the foundation for resilience in the face of changes.

Reflection & Personal Insights

Use the following questions to deepen your self-awareness and consider how you can support yourself through the changes of menopause:

1. What are the symptoms that have impacted me the most?
(Reflect on specific symptoms that have been challenging for you, such as hot flashes or sleep disturbances, and how they have affected your daily life.)

_____

_____

_____

_____

2. What strategies can help me feel more in control of my symptoms?
(Consider any practices mentioned in this chapter—like cooling techniques, setting boundaries, or mindful breathing—that you feel could support you.)

_____

_____

_____

_____

3. How has my perspective on menopause symptoms evolved through this chapter?
(Reflect on any shifts in your mindset, perhaps moving from frustration or confusion to a place of empowerment and understanding.)

_____

_____

_____

_____

_____

4. What role might supplements play in supporting my health and easing symptoms?
(Think about any supplements discussed in this chapter, like magnesium, melatonin, or herbal options, and reflect on whether they might be beneficial additions to your routine.)

_____

_____

_____

_____

_____

5. What small lifestyle change can I make to support my well-being?

(Choose one manageable step, whether it's focusing on sleep, adding a daily mindfulness practice, incorporating gentle movement, or trying a supplement that you can integrate into your life.)

_____

_____

_____

_____

_____

6. What is one affirmation or reminder that can help me stay grounded during challenging moments?

(Consider a phrase that resonates with you, such as "I am resilient" or "I trust my body's wisdom." This can serve as a mental anchor when symptoms arise.)

_____

_____

_____

_____

_____

Use the space on the next page to capture your thoughts, reflections, or anything else that came up for you in this chapter.

Notes

_____

_____

_____

_____

_____

_____

_____

_____

_____

_____

_____

_____

_____

_____

_____

_____

Mindset Check-In:

This is where we pause for a moment. I'd like you to take a deep breath, in through your nose and out through your mouth. You've taken in a lot of information, and it's perfectly okay to feel a little overwhelmed. Take a moment, let everything settle, and give yourself credit for your work. This journey isn't about racing through; it's about allowing each piece to really connect with you, one layer at a time.

In Chapter 1, we started by reshaping how you think about menopause, shifting from old myths to a new, empowering perspective. In Chapter 2, we dove into understanding the three stages of menopause, helping you feel more informed and in control. Then, in Chapter 3, we explored ways to manage those symptoms that can feel so challenging—hot flashes, mood swings, and more—giving you tools to feel more comfortable and confident.

Remember, this isn't just about information—it's about transformation, and that my dear, takes time. So, breathe, acknowledge what you've learned, let it sink in, and know that you're moving forward in a way that honors your pace and your needs. I'm here with you, and together, we'll keep uncovering what you need to thrive in this chapter of life.

When you're ready, we'll continue—taking it one step, one insight at a time.

CHAPTER 4

Prioritizing Nutrition and Hormonal Health

> "Let food be thy medicine and medicine be thy food." — **Hippocrates**

n our last chapter, we touched on the power of nutrition and how the right food choices can make a real difference in managing menopause symptoms. But there's a lot more to dive into here, especially when it comes to choosing foods that truly work with your body. In this chapter, we're going to get more specific—focusing on the types of foods that will support your hormones, help you manage your weight, and keep your energy levels balanced. You'll see how the way we nourish ourselves during menopause can have a tremendous impact on how we feel, day in and day out.

Let's look at how prioritizing protein, selecting quality fats, and being mindful of the right carbs can give your body what it needs to thrive during this stage.

The Power of Protein

Protein is a cornerstone of nutrition and is even more crucial during menopause. We're not just talking about any protein here. For real support, I encourage you to focus on high-quality, nutrient-dense sources: grass-fed meats, wild-caught fish, and pasture-raised poultry. Aim for at least 30 grams of protein per meal. These choices are about more than just flavor; they provide your body with the building blocks needed to maintain muscle mass, support bone health, and manage weight—which is especially important during menopause.

Why prioritize protein? Because it fuels your body in a way that helps it adapt to the changes that come with this stage. As we age, muscle mass naturally declines, and protein becomes essential for preserving that muscle, supporting metabolism, and keeping hunger in check. Try to include a quality protein source at every meal. You'll notice how much more satisfied and balanced you feel when your body is fueled with what it truly needs.

The Importance of Healthy Fats

Hormonal health depends on fats—specifically the right kinds of fats. Our bodies need healthy fats not only to produce hormones but also to support brain function, energy levels, and overall vitality.

I recommend incorporating fats from sources like avocado, olive oil, fatty fish, and butter from grass-fed cows. These aren't just any fats; they're rich in essential fatty acids that help keep you satisfied after meals and offer real nourishment to your cells.

Think of fat as a source of essential fuel. These healthy fats support your body's ability to regulate hormones, stabilize energy levels, and even enhance mental clarity. They're not something to shy away from; rather, they're an ally in navigating menopause and achieving or maintaining a healthy weight with confidence.

Carbs: Choosing the Right Ones

When it comes to carbs, quality matters just as much as quantity, during menopause, choosing carbs that provide nutrients without spiking blood sugar is key. I encourage you to focus on vegetables, particularly cruciferous ones like broccoli, cauliflower, and kale, along with

low-glycemic fruits such as berries. These options provide the energy your body needs without causing the highs and lows that lead to cravings or fatigue.

What's more, these types of carbs are packed with fiber and antioxidants, which help combat oxidative stress—a big bonus for hormonal health. In contrast, avoid grains, nuts, and other high-carb foods that can lead to blood sugar fluctuations and inflammation. Choosing nutrient-dense, low-glycemic carbs gives your body a well-rounded diet that aligns with the balance it needs right now.

Staying Hydrated: The Foundation of Wellness

Hydration might seem basic, but it's one of the most important aspects of being healthy and feeling good day-to-day, especially during menopause. Water plays a huge role in energy levels, skin health, digestion, and even mood. Aim for at least half a gallon a day, and don't overlook the importance of electrolytes—especially when limiting carbs, which can lead to water and electrolyte loss.

While there are many different electrolyte drink mixes out there (LMNT Electrolyte Powder is a popular one), consider adding a pinch of sea salt to your water. This will also help retain the minerals your body needs for balanced hydration. Staying adequately hydrated supports every aspect of your health and helps your body function at its best.

Putting It All Together

With these guidelines, you're not just feeding your body; you're nourishing it in a way that aligns with its unique needs during menopause. This approach isn't about restriction or deprivation—it's about making conscious, intentional choices that honor where you are in life.

Each time you prioritize protein, choose a quality fat, and go for nutrient-dense carbs, you're taking a step towards building a body that feels supported and strong.

By focusing on these key nutritional principles, you're creating a supportive foundation for this stage of life. It's all about choosing foods that work for you, helping you feel energized, balanced, and ready to take on each day.

In the next chapter, we'll dive into the power of exercise and strength training to support you through menopause. From muscle-building workouts to exercises that enhance flexibility and balance, I'll guide you through practical steps to keep your body strong, energized, and resilient. Let's explore how movement can be one of your greatest allies in this new phase of life!

Key Points

- Prioritizing Protein: Protein is essential during menopause for preserving lean muscle mass, supporting bone health, and maintaining a steady metabolism. A protein-rich diet can also help manage weight, keeping you full and energized.

- Choosing the Right Carbohydrates: Focus on nutrient-dense, low-glycemic carbs such as leafy greens, cruciferous vegetables, and berries. These options will help support hormonal balance without causing blood sugar spikes.

- Fats as Essential Fuel: Healthy fats play a vital role in hormone production, brain health, and mood stability. Incorporating sources like avocado, olive oil, fatty fish, and omega-3 supplements can support your body's natural balance during menopause.

- Hydration and Electrolytes: Staying well-hydrated is key to energy, skin health, and digestion. Adding electrolytes, such as a pinch of sea salt, can be particularly helpful, especially on a lower-carb diet.

- Building a Sustainable Plate: A balanced approach to meals—prioritizing protein, the right carbs, and healthy fats—supports a nourishing, menopause-friendly lifestyle without requiring extreme restrictions.

Reflection & Personal Insights

Take a few moments to consider how these nutritional approaches resonate with you and what changes you'd like to explore on your menopause journey. Use these questions to guide your thoughts:

1. How do I feel about making these nutritional shifts during menopause?
(Reflect on whether these changes feel manageable, motivating, or even a bit challenging, and how they align with your current habits and goals.)

_____

_____

_____

_____

2. What challenges or resistance do I feel around prioritizing protein, healthy fats, and nutrient-rich carbs?
(Consider any mental blocks or habits that might be tough to adjust and think about how you can approach these changes with kindness toward yourself.)

_____

_____

_____

_____

3. What small, consistent changes can I make to my diet to support hormonal health?

(Think about simple shifts or adjustments you'd like to try, such as adding more protein at each meal or focusing on low-glycemic carbs.)

_____

_____

_____

_____

_____

4. How might staying hydrated and adding healthy fats improve my daily energy and mood?

(Reflect on your current hydration and fat intake habits and consider how small changes could help you feel more balanced and energized.)

_____

_____

_____

_____

_____

5. What aspect of my eating habits am I most motivated to improve?

(Identify one area where you feel ready to make a positive change, whether it's increasing your protein intake, reducing sugar, or trying new sources of healthy fats.)

Use the space on the next page to capture your thoughts, reflections, or anything else that came up for you in this chapter.

Notes

_____

_____

_____

_____

_____

_____

_____

_____

_____

_____

_____

_____

_____

_____

_____

_____

_____

_____

_____

_____

_____

_____

CHAPTER 5

Exercise and Strength for a New Phase

> "Strength does not come from physical capacity. It comes from an indomitable will."
> — **Mahatma Gandhi**

As we navigate through menopause, maintaining and even building physical strength becomes one of our greatest allies. While the idea of exercise might feel daunting, especially if you're managing new or ongoing symptoms, movement is one of the most effective ways to support your body, mind, and mood. The goal here isn't about reaching peak athletic performance; it's about creating a realistic, empowering approach to exercise that honors where you are and helps you feel strong, resilient, and energized.

In this chapter, we'll explore various forms of exercise and how each type can benefit you during menopause. From strength training to gentle flexibility work, finding the right balance and variety will allow you to build a routine that strengthens your body and mind, supporting you through this transition and beyond.

Why Strength Matters in Menopause

Muscle mass naturally declines with age, and this loss accelerates during menopause due to lower estrogen levels. This decline doesn't just affect strength—it also impacts metabolism, balance, and bone health. The good news? Strength training can counteract these changes, helping you maintain and even gain muscle mass, protect your bones, and support your metabolism.

Strength isn't just physical; it's mental and emotional, too. The empowerment that comes from building strength can influence how we approach the challenges menopause brings. Knowing that you're capable of lifting a weight, completing a workout, or simply moving your body in ways that you may have never moved it before feels powerful, and it can build resilience and confidence in all areas of life.

Building a Well-Rounded Exercise Routine

For an effective and sustainable routine, let's focus on three main categories: strength training, cardiovascular exercise, and flexibility and balance. Each plays a unique role in supporting your body and mind, creating a comprehensive approach that meets your needs at this stage of life.

1. Strength Training: Preserving Muscle and Bone Health

Strength training is essential for building and preserving muscle, maintaining metabolism, and supporting bone density. Aim for two to three sessions per week, focusing on compound movements that engage multiple muscle groups, like squats, lunges, and rows.

If you're new to strength training:

- Start gradually: Begin with body-weight exercises or lighter weights to learn proper form and avoid injury.
- Focus on consistency: It's more beneficial to stay consistent with moderate-intensity workouts than to push yourself too hard and burn out.
- Track your progress: Keep a simple workout log, noting the exercises, weights, and repetitions. Tracking progress can keep you motivated and show you how far you've come.

2. Cardiovascular Exercise: Supporting Heart Health and Energy

Cardio is important for heart health, lung capacity, and overall endurance. You don't need to do intense workouts to see benefits—a brisk walk, cycling, swimming, or dancing can elevate your heart rate and improve circulation.

Aim for 20-30 minutes of moderate cardio, three to four times a week:

- Choose activities you enjoy: The best cardio exercise is the one you'll stick with. If it's fun, you're more likely to keep doing it.
- Mix up the intensity: You can alternate between moderate and more intense days to keep it interesting and support different aspects of cardiovascular health.

- Listen to your body: Cardio should energize you, not exhaust you. Adjust the duration and intensity as needed, especially if you're managing symptoms like fatigue.

3. Flexibility and Balance: Reducing Injury and Enhancing Mobility

Flexibility and balance exercises help prevent injuries, improve posture, and keep your joints healthy. Practices like yoga, Pilates, and Tai Chi can also reduce stress and provide a mental reset.

Consider incorporating 10-15 minutes of flexibility and balance work into your routine daily or a few times a week:

- Stretch with intention: Focus on areas where you feel tightness, such as hips, shoulders, and lower back.
- Practice mindful movement: Slow, controlled movements enhance balance and coordination, supporting overall stability.
- Make it part of your routine: Flexibility and balance work doesn't need to be an intensive session. Gentle stretching in the morning or before bed can make a noticeable difference.

Creating a Routine That Works for You

The key to a sustainable exercise routine is to find what feels right for you. Your needs, energy, and motivation levels will vary, so creating a plan that's flexible and adaptable is essential.

- Set realistic goals: Focus on consistency and gradual progress rather than perfection. Your goal might be to move in some way each day, whether it's a full workout or a gentle stretch.

- Listen to your body: Some days, you might feel ready for a vigorous workout; on others, a gentle walk or stretch may be all you need. Honor where you are each day.
- Celebrate progress: Every step you take is a step forward. Whether it's lifting a heavier weight, walking a little farther, or simply showing up, each achievement is worth celebrating.

Empowering Your Menopause Journey Through Movement

The benefits of exercise during menopause extend beyond physical health. Movement supports mental well-being, reduces stress, boosts mood, and provides a sense of empowerment. When you make movement a regular part of your life, you're nurturing your strength and resilience, setting the foundation for a healthier, more energized you.

In the next chapter, we'll dive into managing stress and sleep—two areas that, like exercise, play a vital role in overall wellness. But for now, let's embrace the power of movement and discover how building strength can positively shape your menopause journey.

Key Points

- Importance of Strength Training: Building muscle during menopause is essential for preserving bone density, metabolism, and overall physical resilience. Strength training two to three times a week is a powerful way to support your body.

- Cardiovascular Health Benefits: Regular cardio enhances heart health, boosts energy, and improves mood. Aim for 20-30 minutes, three to four times a week, focusing on activities you enjoy.
- Flexibility and Balance: Flexibility and balance work, such as yoga or stretching, supports joint health and reduces the risk of injury, helping you move more comfortably and confidently.
- Listening to Your Body: Menopause is a time to prioritize what feels best for you. Honoring your energy levels and adapting your exercise routine to fit how you feel each day leads to sustainable progress.
- Empowerment Through Movement: Exercise during menopause is about more than physical health. It's a journey of building resilience, confidence, and strength to navigate this phase with grace.

Reflection & Personal Insights

Use these questions to reflect on your relationship with movement and how exercise can support you through menopause. Take your time, and remember, there's no "right" answer—this is about what feels best for you.

1. What type of exercise has brought me joy or fulfillment in the past?
(Consider any activities that made you feel strong, energized, or happy. How might you incorporate more of that into your routine now?)

_____

_____

_____

_____

2. How does strength training fit into my life right now?
(Reflect on any thoughts, concerns, or excitement you have about building muscle. What steps could you take to begin or enhance your strength training routine?)

_____

_____

_____

_____

3. What cardio activity could I commit to regularly that feels enjoyable?

(Think about an activity that gets your heart rate up but also feels fun and achievable. How can you make this a consistent part of your routine?)

_____

_____

_____

_____

_____

4. How can flexibility and balance exercises support my overall well-being?

(Identify any areas where you might feel tight, tense, or in need of more flexibility. What type of movement could help you feel more grounded and balanced?)

_____

_____

_____

_____

_____

5. What does a balanced, sustainable exercise routine look like for me?

(Reflect on how you'd like to approach exercise with consistency and self-compassion. Are there ways to adapt your routine to meet your needs and support long-term success?)

Use the space on the next page to capture your thoughts, reflections, or anything else that came up for you in this chapter.

Notes

_____

_____

_____

_____

_____

_____

_____

_____

_____

_____

_____

_____

_____

_____

_____

_____

_____

_____

CHAPTER 6

Finding Balance in Stress and Sleep

"*Almost everything will work again if you unplug it for a few minutes, including you.*"

—Anne Lamott

Stress and sleep are two of the biggest challenges women face during menopause. Hormonal changes can make stress feel more intense and sleep more elusive. It's not just about managing a hectic schedule anymore—your body is navigating an entirely new phase, and it needs rest and calm more than ever. The good news? There are ways to support yourself through these changes and create more ease around both stress and sleep.

In this chapter, we'll dive into the importance of finding balance in stress and sleep, understanding how they're interconnected, and exploring actionable strategies that can make a difference. Just like the other chapters, this isn't about perfection or adding more to your plate—it's about building supportive habits that allow you to feel more grounded and well-rested.

Understanding the Impact of Stress on Menopause

Stress is a part of life, but during menopause, it can feel magnified. The hormonal changes you're experiencing can affect your cortisol levels, sometimes causing you to feel stressed or overwhelmed more easily. And high-stress levels can, in turn, exacerbate menopause symptoms like hot flashes, mood swings, and even weight gain.

The key to managing stress isn't to eliminate it—that's impossible. It's about creating a toolkit of small, daily habits that help you manage it with more ease. Let's look at a few strategies that may help reduce stress naturally:

- Mindful Breathing: A few deep breaths can make a big difference in calming the nervous system. Try inhaling for a count of four, holding for four, and exhaling for six. This can be especially helpful during moments of high stress or when you're feeling overwhelmed.
- Setting Boundaries: Learning to say no and protect your time is an act of self-care
- Think about what truly needs your attention and let go of things that don't serve you. Boundaries can be

empowering, helping you preserve energy for what matters most.

- Prioritizing Joy: It's easy to let joyful activities slide when life gets busy, but they're actually essential. Small moments of joy—a walk outside, a favorite song, or a good laugh—help reset your stress levels and remind you of what feels good.

By weaving these simple practices into your day, you can create moments of calm that help regulate your body's response to stress, making the menopause journey smoother.

The Essential Role of Sleep in Menopause

Sleep often becomes challenging during menopause. You might find yourself waking up in the middle of the night, struggling to fall back asleep, or feeling tired even after a full night in bed.

Poor sleep doesn't just leave you feeling groggy—it affects everything from your mood to your metabolism and even your immune system. In other words, quality sleep is essential.

Here are some practical ways to support better sleep:

- Establish a Calming Evening Routine: Think of it as a wind-down ritual. Turn off screens, dim the lights, and engage in a relaxing activity like reading or taking a warm bath. This can signal to your body that it's time for rest.
- Create a Sleep-Friendly Environment: A cool, dark, quiet room can do wonders for sleep quality. Consider blackout curtains, a fan, or white noise to create a space that encourages uninterrupted rest.

- Limit Stimulants in the Afternoon: Caffeine and alcohol can interfere with sleep quality, especially when consumed later in the day. If you're finding it hard to stay asleep, consider cutting back on stimulants after lunchtime.

- Consider Natural Sleep Aids: Certain natural supplements may offer extra support for restful sleep. Melatonin (3-5 mg about 30-60 minutes before bed) can help reset your sleep-wake cycle, while magnesium (200-400 mg) can help relax your muscles. GABA (750 mg) may also promote relaxation. Always check with a healthcare provider before trying new supplements to ensure they're right for you.

The Connection Between Stress and Sleep

Stress and sleep are closely linked; one affects the other. When you're stressed, it can be harder to fall asleep or stay asleep. And when you don't sleep well, you're more prone to stress, creating a cycle that can feel challenging to break.

Understanding this connection can be empowering because it means small changes in one area can positively affect the other. By working on stress-reduction practices during the day and creating a relaxing nighttime routine, you're supporting both areas simultaneously. This isn't about making drastic changes; it's about small, manageable shifts that support your well-being.

Practical Tools for Balancing Stress and Sleep

Finding balance in these areas doesn't have to be overwhelming. It's about discovering what feels most supportive and realistic for you. Here's a quick list of tools that might help:

- Practice Gratitude: Take a few moments each day to reflect on what you're grateful for. Gratitude can shift your perspective and help you feel more positive, even in challenging times.
- Mindful Movement: Gentle exercise, like walking or yoga, can be an excellent way to release stress and promote better sleep. Find movement that feels good for you and fits into your lifestyle.
- Stay Connected: Reach out to friends or loved ones. Talking about your experiences can help you feel more supported and less alone, which is essential for emotional well-being.
- Limit Blue Light Exposure: Avoid screens for at least an hour before bed. Blue light from phones, tablets, and computers can interfere with the production of melatonin, the hormone that regulates sleep.

These practices are small, but they add up over time, helping you feel more balanced and in control. Menopause may bring its own unique set of challenges, but with a supportive approach to stress and sleep, you're building a strong foundation for resilience.

As we move into the next chapter, we'll dive into the power of building a resilient mindset—one that allows you to handle the ups and downs of menopause with confidence and inner strength.

Key Points

- Stress Management is Essential: Stress can amplify menopause symptoms, making it crucial to integrate stress-management practices like mindful breathing, setting boundaries, and prioritizing joyful moments.

- Prioritizing Quality Sleep: Quality sleep is essential for hormonal health, emotional well-being, and energy. Simple steps like a calming evening routine and a sleep-friendly environment can improve sleep quality.
- The Interplay Between Stress and Sleep: Recognizing the connection between stress and sleep can empower you to make small adjustments in both areas, leading to better overall balance.
- Practical Tools for Balance: Practical habits like gratitude, gentle movement, and limiting blue light exposure can support stress reduction and improve sleep.
- Exploring Natural Sleep Aids: Supplements like melatonin, magnesium, and GABA (with guidance from a healthcare provider) can offer additional support for restful sleep.

Reflection & Personal Insights

Take a moment to reflect on how stress and sleep show up in your life and consider how small adjustments could help. Use these prompts to guide your thoughts.

1. How has stress affected me, and what triggers seem to impact me most
(Reflect on any patterns you've noticed and consider which stress-management techniques could help you feel more balanced.)

_____

_____

_____

_____

2. What sleep challenges have I experienced, and how have they impacted my mood or energy?
(Think about the quality of your sleep and whether certain routines or habits could support better rest.)

_____

_____

_____

_____

_____

3. Which stress-reduction strategies feel most doable for me right now?

(Consider small practices, like breathing exercises or prioritizing joyful moments, that you could try on a regular basis.)

_____

_____

_____

_____

_____

4. What adjustments could help me create a more restful sleep environment?

(Think about how you can optimize your bedtime routine and sleep environment to support relaxation and deep sleep.)

_____

_____

_____

_____

_____

_____

5. How can I show myself more compassion in managing stress and sleep?

(Reflect on the importance of being kind to yourself in this journey, allowing for flexibility and understanding as you make changes.)

_____

_____

_____

_____

_____

_____

_____

_____

_____

_____

_____

_____

_____

_____

Use the space on the next page to capture your thoughts, reflections, or anything else that came up for you in this chapter.

Notes

Mindset Check-In:

Let's take a moment again to pause, breathe, and let everything settle. You're doing an incredible job of diving deep, and these last few chapters were no small feat. Let's acknowledge the journey you're on and the insights you're gathering along the way.

In Chapter 4, we focused on building a lifestyle that truly supports your body through nutrition—understanding the power of prioritizing protein, healthy fats, and nourishing carbs that work with you, not against you. In Chapter 5, we discussed the importance of strength and movement, finding a rhythm of exercise that fuels your energy and keeps you feeling strong. In Chapter 6, we explored stress and sleep, two pillars of wellness that often go hand-in-hand, giving you tools to create a balanced, restful space for yourself.

It's a lot to take in, and it's okay to feel like you're still figuring out what fits best for you. The beautiful thing is that you're building this path step by step, each chapter helping you to shape a stronger, more resilient version of yourself. Let yourself feel proud of the work you've done so far, and remember—this is your journey, unfolding exactly as it should.

When you're ready, we'll continue on, embracing each layer of growth as it comes.

CHAPTER 7

Building a Resilient Mindset

> *"The mind is everything. What you think, you become." — **Buddha***

As you go through menopause, it's easy to feel like everything is changing faster than you can keep up. Your body is going through so much, and sometimes it can feel overwhelming, especially if you're also dealing with unexpected emotions. But here's the thing: resilience is your greatest strength during this time, and building a resilient mindset will give you the tools to navigate menopause with grace, strength, and self-compassion.

Think of resilience as your inner strength, a source of calm and courage that you can rely on. It's about knowing that, no matter what menopause brings, you have the power to face it with confidence. I know first hand that this isn't always easy, but resilience is ksomething you can build, and it starts with how you speak to yourself, how you approach challenges, and how willing you are to believe in your ability to adapt and thrive.

In this chapter, let's talk about what it means to build a resilient mindset and how you can cultivate a sense of calm, strength, and confidence, even when things feel tough. You are stronger than you know, and you're capable of weathering this storm—and coming out stronger on the other side.

Shifting Your Self-Talk

One of the first steps in building resilience is becoming aware of your inner dialogue—the things you say to yourself, especially during moments of stress or self-doubt. If you're constantly being hard on yourself, it's time to shift that self-talk to something kinder and more supportive. Imagine talking to a friend who's going through the same thing. You wouldn't be harsh or critical; you'd be encouraging and understanding. So why not offer yourself that same compassion?

When you catch yourself thinking, "I can't handle this" or "I'm not strong enough," pause and replace those thoughts with something more positive and empowering. Tell yourself, "I'm learning and growing through this," or "I'm doing the best I can, and that's enough." These small shifts in how you talk to yourself can make a huge difference in building resilience.

Embracing Flexibility and Adaptability

Resilience isn't about being unbreakable; it's about being flexible, like a tree that bends in the wind but doesn't snap. Menopause may require you to adapt in ways you hadn't anticipated, whether that's in your daily routines, relationships, or how you take care of your body.

Embracing flexibility—being open to change and willing to try new things—allows you to move through these shifts with greater ease and grace.

Consider viewing this time as an opportunity for growth rather than something to "get through." Each challenge is a chance to learn more about yourself and discover strengths you didn't know you had. And remember, resilience doesn't mean you have to handle everything alone. It's okay to ask for help or lean on others when you need it.

Focusing on Gratitude and Positivity

Gratitude is a powerful tool for resilience. When we take a moment to focus on what's going right, rather than only on the challenges, it helps us stay grounded and positive. This doesn't mean ignoring the difficulties but choosing to also notice the good moments—the days when you feel more energized, the support of loved ones, the small victories.

Try keeping a gratitude journal or simply taking a few minutes each day to think about three things you're grateful for. Practicing gratitude helps shift your focus from frustration to appreciation and gives you a renewed sense of strength to face the ups and downs of menopause.

Building Your Support Network

Resilience is often strengthened by the people we surround ourselves with. Whether it's family, friends, a support group, or other women going through menopause, having a network of people who understand and support you is invaluable. They can offer encouragement, share in your triumphs, and remind you that you're not alone.

If you don't have a strong support network right now, consider joining a community, either in-person or online, where you can connect with others on this journey. Sharing your experiences and listening to others can be a great way to build resilience and feel connected.

Let's end this chapter with a reminder: Resilience isn't about never struggling; it's about learning how to navigate those struggles with strength and grace. You're already resilient just by being here, willing to explore these questions and do this work. Remember, you're not alone, and you have everything within you to handle this stage with courage and confidence.

Key Points

- Resilience as Inner Strength: Resilience is about embracing your inner strength and using it to face the challenges of menopause with confidence and grace. It's a skill that grows over time, helping you navigate changes with calm and courage.

- Self-Talk as a Tool for Resilience: How you speak to yourself matters. Shifting negative self-talk to something kinder and more supportive helps build resilience and empowers you to believe in your own strength.
- Flexibility and Adaptability: Building resilience means being flexible and open to adapting as menopause brings changes. This adaptability is what helps you move through challenges without feeling overwhelmed.
- Gratitude as a Foundation for Positivity: Practicing gratitude daily shifts your focus from what's difficult to what's good, grounding you in positivity and making it easier to stay resilient.
- Strengthening Your Support Network: Having a support system—whether friends, family, or a community—provides encouragement and reminds you that you're not alone on this journey.

Reflection & Personal Insights

Reflect on how you can cultivate resilience in your life during this time. Use these prompts to dive deeper and explore ways to strengthen your inner resources.

1. What does resilience mean to me?
(Reflect on your personal definition of resilience and how it plays a role in your life.)

_____

_____

_____

_____

_____

2. How can I improve my self-talk?
(Consider the things you often say to yourself, especially during difficult moments. How could you shift this self-talk to be more encouraging and supportive?)

_____

_____

_____

_____

_____

3. In what areas can I be more flexible and open to change?
(Think about the areas where you might be holding onto rigidity. How could embracing flexibility help you move through menopause more smoothly?)

_____

_____

_____

_____

_____

_____

4. What are three things I'm grateful for today?
(List three things that bring you joy or peace today. This simple practice can shift your perspective and build a foundation of positivity.)

_____

_____

_____

_____

_____

_____

5. Who in my life can I lean on for support?

(Identify people who can support you through this journey. If you don't have a strong network, think about ways you could start building one.)

_____

_____

_____

_____

_____

_____

_____

_____

_____

_____

_____

_____

_____

Use the space on the next page to capture your thoughts, reflections, or anything else that came up for you in this chapter.

Notes

_____

_____

_____

_____

_____

_____

_____

_____

_____

_____

_____

_____

_____

_____

_____

_____

_____

_____

_____

CHAPTER 8

Embracing Self-Care and Setting Boundaries

> *"You yourself, as much as anybody in the entire universe, deserve your love and affection."* — **Buddha**

You've made it so far on this journey, and you're doing the work to better understand yourself and navigate menopause with strength. Now, it's time to talk about something that many of us often overlook: self-care and setting boundaries. These two practices are the foundation of taking care of yourself, especially during a season as transformative as menopause.

Self-care isn't just a buzzword—it's a form of respect for yourself. It's about listening to your body, honoring your needs, and allowing yourself the space to recharge. Boundaries, on the other hand, are like the protective walls that keep your energy and well-being safe. Together, they form a powerful toolkit that helps you show up for yourself and, ultimately, for those you love.

But here's the challenge: for many of us, prioritizing self-care and setting boundaries doesn't come naturally. We're used to putting others first, often feeling guilty if we take time for ourselves or say "no" when we need to. But here's what I want you to know—you deserve that time, and you deserve those boundaries. You have permission to put yourself first.

In this chapter, let's explore what self-care can look like for you, how to create boundaries that feel empowering, and why these practices are essential, especially at this stage of life.

Defining Self-Care on Your Terms

When we talk about self-care, it doesn't have to mean bubble baths and spa days—unless, of course, that's what fills you up! Self-care is deeply personal, and it's about finding practices that genuinely nourish your body, mind, and spirit.

Ask yourself: what does self-care look like for me? Maybe it's spending time outdoors, reading a good book, taking a quiet moment with a cup of tea, or even setting aside time each day to meditate or journal. It doesn't have to be elaborate or time-consuming. True self-care is about consistency and intention—finding small moments in your day that remind you that you matter.

This is your invitation to make self-care a non-negotiable part of your routine. These little moments of care add up and send a powerful message: you're worth taking care of.

Setting Boundaries with Confidence

Boundaries are one of the greatest acts of self-love, yet they're also one of the hardest. Saying "no" can feel uncomfortable, especially if you're used to being the one who says "yes" to everyone else's needs. But here's the truth: every time you say "yes" to something that doesn't align with your well-being, you're saying "no" to yourself.

Boundaries are about protecting your time, your energy, and your peace. Think about areas in your life where you might be overextending yourself or feeling drained. Maybe it's saying yes to too many commitments, answering calls when you need quiet time, or taking on tasks that aren't truly yours to carry. Boundaries are about deciding what you're willing to accept and where you need to draw the line.

And remember, setting boundaries doesn't make you selfish—it makes you stronger. It allows you to show up fully for the things that truly matter, without feeling depleted or resentful.

Practicing Guilt-Free Self-Care

One of the biggest challenges I hear from women is the guilt that comes with self-care and setting boundaries. It's that nagging feeling that you're doing something "wrong" by putting yourself first. But let's flip the script on that. Taking care of yourself doesn't mean you're neglecting others; it means you're creating a stronger, healthier version of yourself for everyone around you.

Think of self-care as a gift you give not just to yourself, but to those you love. When you're well-rested, grounded, and at peace, you can bring your best self to every part of your life. So, when those feelings of guilt creep in, remind yourself that this isn't about indulgence—it's about resilience and well-being.

Creating a Self-Care Routine That Works for You

Building a self-care routine doesn't have to be complicated. Start with something small and build from there. Here are a few ideas to get you started:

- Morning Moments: Begin your day with a small ritual that grounds you, like stretching, journaling, or simply enjoying a quiet cup of coffee.
- Movement: Find a form of exercise you enjoy, whether it's walking, yoga, or dancing. Moving your body is one of the best ways to take care of yourself physically and mentally.
- Mindfulness Practice: Take five to ten minutes a day to check in with yourself. This could be through meditation, deep breathing, or simply sitting quietly and letting your thoughts settle.
- End-of-Day Wind Down: Set aside time each evening to unwind. This could mean reading, soaking in a warm bath, or writing down a few things you're grateful for from the day.

Remember, there's no right or wrong way to do this. Self-care is about experimenting and discovering what nourishes you.

Embracing Boundaries with Grace

Setting boundaries is a skill, and like any skill, it takes practice. Start small and be gentle with yourself. You might feel uncomfortable at first, but with each boundary you set, you'll start to feel a little stronger and more in control.

When you set a boundary, remember that you don't owe anyone an explanation. A simple, kind, "I'm sorry, I can't commit to that right now" is enough. Trust that the people who care about you will respect your needs, and let go of the rest.

Let's end with a reminder: self-care and boundaries aren't about building walls or being selfish; they're about creating a space for you to thrive. You're giving yourself permission to be well, to be whole, and to embrace this time of life with strength and peace. And that's something worth celebrating.

Key Points

- Self-Care as a Priority: Self-care isn't selfish; it's essential. By taking time for yourself, you're investing in your health, happiness, and ability to show up fully for those you love.
- Boundaries as Protection for Well-Being: Boundaries protect your time, energy, and peace. They're a form of self-respect and allow you to give your best self to the things and people that truly matter.
- Letting Go of Guilt: Guilt has no place in self-care. Embracing self-care and setting boundaries isn't a luxury—it's a necessity that benefits everyone around you.

- Creating a Personalized Self-Care Routine: Self-care doesn't have to be elaborate. Building small, consistent practices into your day can have a powerful impact on your overall well-being.
- Practicing and Honoring Boundaries: Boundaries are a skill that takes time to develop, but each boundary you set strengthens your sense of self and protects your energy.

Reflection & Personal Insights

Take some time to explore your thoughts and feelings about self-care and boundaries. Use these prompts to guide your reflection:

1. How can I start seeing self-care as a form of self-respect?
(Reflect on why self-care has been challenging and what needs to shift to see it as something you deserve.)

_____

_____

_____

_____

_____

2. What boundaries would feel empowering to set?
(Think about areas in your life where boundaries could protect your peace and well-being. List one or two boundaries you'd like to create.)

_____

_____

_____

_____

_____

3. How can I release the guilt around putting myself first?
(Consider where the guilt comes from and what you need to let go
of to feel more comfortable embracing self-care and boundaries.)

_____
_____
_____
_____
_____
_____

4. What small self-care practice am I willing to try this week?
(Pick one self-care activity you can start doing regularly, even if it's
just five minutes a day.)

_____
_____
_____
_____
_____
_____
_____

5. Who supports my boundaries, and how can I lean into that support?

(Identify people who encourage your self-care and boundaries. Think about how you can draw strength from that support.)

_____

_____

_____

_____

_____

_____

_____

_____

_____

_____

_____

_____

_____

Use the space on the next page to capture your thoughts, reflections, or anything else that came up for you in this chapter.

Notes

CHAPTER 9

Navigating Relationships and Finding Support

> *"Surround yourself with only people who are going to lift you higher."* **— Oprah Winfrey**

Menopause is a journey that brings a lot of changes, both inside and out. And as you go through these changes, relationships can be one of the most meaningful sources of support—or they can be a source of stress. Relationships with partners, family, friends, and even coworkers can feel a little different during this time, and it's natural to feel both closer to some people and more distant from others. This chapter is all about helping you navigate those relationships with intention and finding the support that truly nurtures you.

You don't have to go through menopause alone. Having people around you who understand, respect, and encourage you can make a world of difference. And yet, it can sometimes feel challenging to explain what you're going through or ask for the support you need. My hope is that by the end of this chapter, you'll feel empowered to communicate openly with those close to you, deepen the relationships that bring you joy, and surround yourself with a supportive community that lifts you up.

Redefining Relationships During Menopause

One of the things that makes menopause unique is how it changes our sense of self—and with it, the way we relate to others. This is a time of self-discovery, and as you get to know this new version of yourself, you may find that some relationships evolve naturally. Perhaps you're craving deeper connections, or maybe you're realizing that certain relationships no longer serve you in the way they once did.

Remember, it's okay for relationships to shift and change. This season of life is a chance to redefine who you want around you, to strengthen the relationships that nourish you, and to gently release those that may be weighing you down.

Communicating Your Needs Openly

Menopause can be difficult for others to fully understand, especially if they haven't experienced it themselves. Partners, family members, or friends may want to support you but aren't sure how. This is where open communication becomes essential.

Start by sharing what you're experiencing in a way that feels authentic to you. You don't have to go into every detail—just enough for them to understand what you're going through. For example, you might explain that some days you need a little extra patience or that sometimes you just need a quiet moment to yourself.

One of the most empowering things you can do is communicate your needs without guilt. Asking for understanding, patience, or support isn't a burden; it's a way of inviting those you care about to be part of your journey. And the more open you are, the more likely it is that they'll respond with compassion.

Strengthening Bonds with Empathy and Understanding

Menopause can deepen connections, especially when there's mutual empathy and understanding. Sometimes, it's as simple as having a heartfelt conversation or finding shared activities that make you feel close to those you care about. Spending time with friends or family members who accept you as you are can be incredibly healing, especially when you're feeling vulnerable.

Take time to nurture these bonds. Let your loved ones know you value their support, and show gratitude for the ways they stand by you. Little gestures—like a text to check in, a shared meal, or a quick phone call—can mean the world in maintaining and strengthening these connections.

Setting Boundaries with Grace

Just as important as nurturing healthy relationships is setting boundaries with those that feel draining or unfulfilling. Menopause is a time when your emotional and physical energy might feel more limited, and it's okay to protect that energy.

Maybe there are people who don't understand what you're going through or who bring negativity into your life. You have every right to set boundaries with these individuals. Boundaries are about creating a safe space where you can focus on your well-being. Whether it's limiting time with certain people or simply saying "no" to things that don't serve you, these boundaries allow you to show up for the relationships that truly matter.

Seeking Out Supportive Communities

Sometimes, the most meaningful support comes from others who are on a similar path. Finding a community of women who are also navigating menopause can provide a sense of comfort and camaraderie that's hard to find elsewhere. Whether it's an online forum like Meetup, a local support group, or even a close friend going through similar changes, these connections remind you that you're not alone.

Consider joining a menopause support group or finding an online community where you can share your experiences and hear from others who understand. These spaces can be incredibly validating, offering a chance to learn, laugh, and even find a little lightheartedness in the midst of it all.

Embracing the Power of Connection

As you navigate this journey, remember that relationships and support networks are there to enrich your life, not drain it. Surround yourself with people who lift you up, who understand that you're going through a period of transformation, and who respect the boundaries you set. These connections are a powerful source of resilience, comfort, and joy as you move forward.

Remember, the relationships you nurture and the support you seek are there to make this journey lighter, not heavier. Embrace those who walk alongside you, and let go of what no longer serves you. You deserve relationships that enrich your life, especially now.

In the next chapter, we'll bring together all that we've explored and work on creating your own personal blueprint for thriving through menopause and beyond. You're not just surviving this season— you're building a life that feels empowering, supported, and deeply fulfilling.

Key Points

- Redefining Relationships: Menopause can change how you relate to others, allowing you to redefine which relationships support your well-being and which may need gentle boundaries.
- Open Communication: Honest communication with loved ones fosters empathy and understanding, making it easier for them to support you.

- Strengthening Connections: Building bonds through empathy and shared activities helps deepen relationships that bring joy and comfort during menopause.
- Setting Boundaries: Protecting your emotional and physical energy with boundaries allows you to focus on relationships that are nurturing and positive.
- Seeking Community Support: Connecting with other women on the menopause journey offers camaraderie, validation, and a reminder that you're not alone.

Reflection & Personal Insights

Take some time to reflect on your relationships and the support networks in your life. These questions can help you explore ways to strengthen connections that support you and set boundaries where needed.

1. Which relationships in my life feel most nourishing right now?
(Consider the people who make you feel seen, understood, and supported. How can you deepen these connections?)

_____

_____

_____

_____

2. How can I communicate my needs more openly with those close to me?
(Think about any specific needs you have and how you might share these with loved ones in an honest, gentle way.)

_____

_____

_____

_____

_____

3. Are there any relationships where I need to set clear boundaries?

(Reflect on any connections that feel draining or unfulfilling and how you can protect your energy through boundaries.)

_____

_____

_____

_____

_____

4. Where might I find additional support or community?

(Consider whether a support group, online community, or friend might provide the camaraderie you need during this season.)

_____

_____

_____

_____

_____

5. What small actions can I take to nurture my relationships?
(Identify a few small gestures, like checking in with a friend or planning a get-together, to keep your connections strong and supportive.)

_____

_____

_____

_____

_____

_____

_____

_____

_____

_____

_____

_____

_____

Use the space on the next page to capture your thoughts, reflections, or anything else that came up for you in this chapter.

Notes

Mindset Check-In:

This is your last check-in. Take a deep, steadying breath. You've journeyed through so much and should be incredibly proud of the time, thought, and heart you've invested in this process. It's not always easy to pause, reflect, and answer thought-provoking questions with honesty, but here you are, having navigated each layer with grace and resilience. Give yourself a moment to recognize the depth of what you've accomplished.

In Chapter 7, we explored the power of a resilient mindset, laying a foundation to support you through every phase of change. You learned that building inner strength is just as vital as any physical practice. In Chapter 8, we dived into the art of self-care and the importance of setting boundaries. Self-care isn't just a treat; it's essential. Setting boundaries honors your energy and gives you the space to prioritize what truly matters. Then, in Chapter 9, we looked at relationships and support, recognizing that no journey is meant to be traveled alone, and remember, you are not alone. You gained insight into finding strength in connection and embracing the support that surrounds you.

You've done the work—you've reflected, set intentions, and gained valuable awareness about yourself and this chapter of life. It's okay if you feel a mix of emotions right now. Transformation doesn't happen overnight, and the steps you've taken are laying the groundwork for continued growth and confidence.

As we move into Chapter 10, we're going to put it all together. This is where the deep dive transitions into action, where everything you've learned becomes part of a clear, empowering path forward. You've prepared yourself for this moment by understanding your needs, your boundaries, and your inner strength. Now, you'll be equipped to integrate these insights into your daily life, taking all of the knowledge, compassion, and resilience you've cultivated and applying it in ways that support your health, happiness, and well-being.

So let's step forward with confidence, knowing that you are ready. The next phase is about putting it all together—and you have every tool you need to do just that.

CHAPTER 10

Putting It All Together

Your Blueprint for Thriving Through Menopause

> *"The journey of a thousand miles begins with a single step."* — **Lao Tzu**

Here we are, at the end of the journey we've taken together through these pages.mkmy;j You've explored what it means to go through menopause, learned about the stages, navigated symptoms, built resilience, prioritized self-care, and set boundaries. Each chapter was designed to help you get in touch with what your body, mind, and soul need during this time. And all of this matters—because real change happens when you're in tune with yourself, not just following a checklist of things to do.

Menopause is a journey of transformation, one that affects every part of who you are. It's about more than just what you eat or how you exercise; it's about knowing yourself deeply, honoring your needs, and creating a life that feels balanced and fulfilling. So before we jump into any rapid weight loss plan, it's essential to understand that physical changes are only part of the picture.

Finding Your Foundation

Throughout this book, we've taken a close look at the many areas of life that menopause touches. Nutrition, exercise, sleep, mindset, and relationships—each play a role in how you feel and how you approach change. These aren't isolated pieces; they're interconnected. When you're clear on your boundaries, manage stress, and prioritize sleep, everything else can fall into place. Building a strong foundation is about creating harmony between these parts so that when you're ready to focus on weight loss or fitness, you have the support and structure you need to stay consistent.

Why It's Not Just About the Weight

I know that weight loss may be one of, or quite possibly, your only goals in reading this book, and I fully understand why. For many of us, gaining weight feels like it's out of our control, especially during menopause. But let me tell you this: sustainable weight loss isn't just about what's on your plate or how much you exercise. It's about feeling good in your own skin, about having the energy to do what you love, and about being confident in the choices you make for your body.

That's why I included all the chapters leading up to this. We had to dive into where you are mentally and emotionally, how you feel about your body, and what you need for yourself at this stage of life. Setting boundaries, managing stress, and focusing on self-care are just as important as any workout or meal plan because they lay the groundwork for real, lasting change. When your mind is ready, your body is far more likely to follow.

The Mindset Shift: Preparing for Lifestyle Changes

As you think about this 10-day program, I want you to consider it as a stepping stone, not an end goal. This isn't just about a quick fix or shedding a few pounds; it's about giving you the tools and motivation to build a lifestyle that feels sustainable and aligned with your needs. Real change takes time, patience, and compassion for yourself. And that compassion includes being ready mentally to commit to these changes.

So, before starting this program, take a moment to check in with yourself. Are you feeling prepared? Do you feel supported? Are you excited about this next step? This isn't about perfection—it's about feeling ready to make choices that honor your well-being.

The Physical Component: A 10-Day Jumpstart

With this foundation in place, we're ready to get into the physical component: a 10-day exercise and meal plan that's designed to kick-start your journey. This program is all about balance— nourishing your body with high-quality foods and energizing it with movement that feels good. It's not about restriction or overdoing it;

ls

it's about fueling your body and enjoying the process. Each day will include a structured meal plan and a gentle, achievable workout tailored to give you the boost you need to feel strong, confident, and empowered.

Moving Forward

As you start this 10-day program, remember that you have everything within you to make it a success. You've done the work to prepare mentally and emotionally, and now it's time to put it all into practice. This journey is yours, and I'm here cheering you on every step of the way. You've got the tools, the knowledge, and the confidence to move forward, creating a life that truly feels good.

In the end, menopause is about so much more than symptoms or weight—it's about reconnecting with yourself, embracing each new chapter, and finding joy in the process. This is your time to thrive, and I'm honored to have been a part of this journey with you.

Key Points

- Building a Foundation: A balanced approach that includes nutrition, sleep, stress management, and mindset creates a strong base for any lifestyle change.
- The Whole-Body Connection: Sustainable change comes from aligning mind and body, not just focusing on diet and exercise.
- Weight as Part of the Bigger Picture: Weight loss can be a goal, but it's one part of a holistic journey that includes mental and emotional well-being.

- Preparedness for Change: The 10-day program is designed to help you start with intention, using everything you've learned to build momentum.
- Empowerment Through Self-Care: Each step in this journey is about honoring your body, mind, and spirit—taking action from a place of self-love.

Reflection & Personal Insights

Take a moment to reflect on how far you've come in this journey and where you're headed next. These questions can help you center yourself as you begin the 10-day program.

1. How has my understanding of menopause evolved through this journey?
(Reflect on any shifts in perspective you've had about what menopause means and how it affects you.)

_____

_____

_____

_____

_____

2. What areas of my life have I strengthened or clarified?
(Think about specific changes you've made in areas like self-care, boundaries, or mindset, and how they've impacted you.)

_____

_____

_____

_____

_____

3. How do I feel about starting the 10-day program?

(Consider if you're feeling mentally and physically ready to begin, and what adjustments you might need for a successful start.)

_____

_____

_____

_____

_____

_____

_____

4. What are my goals for this next phase?

(Identify one or two personal goals for the 10-day program, whether it's feeling more energized, reconnecting with exercise, or improving your eating habits.)

_____

_____

_____

_____

_____

_____

_____

5. What positive affirmations or reminders can I use to stay motivated?

(Create a simple affirmation to keep you focused and inspired, such as "I am capable and prepared to honor my health and well-being.")

_____

_____

_____

_____

_____

_____

_____

_____

_____

_____

_____

_____

Use the space on the next page to capture your thoughts, reflections, or anything else that came up for you in this chapter.

Notes

WELCOME

to Your 10-Day Rapid Weight Loss Program

Congratulations on reaching this part of your journey! By now, you've gained valuable insights, built resilience, and set boundaries that empower you to take control of your health and

well-being. This 10-day rapid weight loss program is designed to give you a strong foundation, combining a carefully crafted meal plan and an empowering exercise plan to support your goals and help you feel your best.

This program isn't about restriction or perfection—it's about creating balance, building momentum, and finding joy in nourishing and moving your body. Whether your focus is on shedding weight, boosting your energy, or simply feeling more like yourself, these next 10 days are designed to help you jumpstart your journey with confidence and clarity.

Nourish Your Body

The 10-day meal plan is crafted with simplicity and balance in mind, focusing on nutrient-dense foods that energize and satisfy. Each meal is thoughtfully designed to provide the right mix of protein, healthy fats, and low-glycemic carbs to support hormonal health and promote rapid weight loss—all while being easy to prepare and enjoy.

You also have access to a **Grocery List** and **Approved Foods List** to make shopping and planning a breeze. Feel free to explore the recipes, savor the meals, and even swap out options to suit your preferences. Flexibility is key!

Your Flexible Options

If you're short on time or feel like mixing things up, you're welcome to replace any meal with a **Grass-Fed Beef Protein Smoothie** or an **Egg White Protein Smoothie**. These smoothies are packed with nutrients and provide a quick, easy alternative while keeping you on track. You can also use the **Approved Foods List** to create your own balanced meals. This plan is adaptable to your lifestyle and preferences while still delivering results.

Move with Intention

The exercise component of this program is designed to complement your nutritional efforts, helping you build strength, boost energy, and feel empowered. It incorporates a mix of:

- **Strength Training** to preserve muscle, support metabolism, and enhance bone health.

- **Cardio** to boost heart health, improve stamina, and release endorphins for a natural mood lift.
- **Flexibility and Balance Work** like yoga or stretching to reduce tension, increase mobility, and prevent injury.

A Flexible Approach

Each workout includes guidance but allows for flexibility to match your body's needs. Start each session by checking in with yourself—how do you feel today? Whether you're ready for a challenge or need a lighter movement day, this plan is here to support you without adding stress or pressure.

Helpful Tips for Success

To make the most of your 10-day journey, here are a few tips to set you up for success:

1. Listen to Your Hunger Cues

If you're not hungry first thing in the morning, it's okay to push breakfast to a later time. Remember, "breakfast" is simply breaking your overnight fast—it doesn't have to be early in the day.

2. Finish Meals by 7 pm

Ending your meals by 7 pm gives your body time to digest before bed, supporting better sleep and weight management.

3. Stay Hydrated

Aim to drink half your body weight in ounces of water daily. Hydration supports digestion, energy levels, and weight loss.

4. Prioritize Protein

Each meal includes high-quality protein, essential for maintaining muscle, supporting metabolism, and keeping you satisfied.

5. Incorporate Movement

Find ways to move daily—whether it's walking, strength training, or stretching. Consistent activity enhances fat-burning, boosts mood, and supports overall well-being.

6. Practice Mindful Eating

Eat slowly and savor each bite, tuning into hunger and fullness cues.

7. Focus on Rest and Recovery

Quality sleep is essential for weight loss and overall health. Aim for 7-8 hours of restful sleep each night.

8. Plan Ahead

Take a few minutes each day to prepare for your meals and workouts. A little planning goes a long way toward staying on track.

Continuing Beyond the 10 Days

By the end of the 10 days, you'll have established a solid routine and built momentum. If you'd like to continue, you can repeat the program as many times as needed or use the **Approved Foods List** to create your own meals.

For those looking to dive deeper, the book includes a **14-Day Sample Exercise Plan** to guide you through a structured continuation of movement. You also have access to additional tracking and journaling pages to extend your progress.

For a more comprehensive approach, consider my **Menopause Weight Loss Blueprint**—a done-for-you program that takes an even deeper dive into:

- BHRT and hormonal health.
- Bone density and strength-building strategies.
- Advanced intermittent fasting techniques.
- Long-term weight management and lifestyle tools.

This program offers everything you need to navigate menopause and weight loss with ease and confidence.

Let's Get Started

This 10-day plan is your first step in a journey that's all about you— your health, your strength, and your well-being. Let's move forward with confidence, knowing you're equipped with the tools to succeed.

Here's to a fulfilling and transformative 10 days and beyond!

10-DAY

Rapid Weight Loss
Exercise Plan

During these 10 days, you'll be free to choose different activities each day, combining strength training, cardio, and flexibility exercises in any order that feels right for you. The key is to engage in one type of movement each day so you're consistently building strength, stamina, and flexibility.

For the Next 10 Days: Choose One Activity Each Day

For each day of the 10-Day Rapid Weight Loss Plan, select one of the three types of exercise below:

1. Strength Training: Focus on either upper or lower body.
2. Cardio: Aim for 20 minutes of steady-state cardio.
3. Flexibility: Incorporate yoga, Pilates, or simple stretching.

For instance, your 10-day exercise schedule could look something like this:

- Day 1: Strength Training (Upper Body)
- Day 2: Cardio
- Day 3: Flexibility
- Day 4: Strength Training (Lower Body)
- Day 5: Cardio
- Day 6: Flexibility
- Day 7: Strength Training (Upper Body)
- Day 8: Cardio
- Day 9: Flexibility
- Day 10: Strength Training (Lower Body)

By the end of these 10 days, you'll have laid a strong foundation for a routine that not only builds momentum but sets the tone for lasting change. Following this structure will help you stay active, motivated, and confident as you move forward. So stay consistent and keep progressing toward your health and weight-loss goals.

Long-Term Exercise Routine: Moving Forward

Once you've completed the 10-day plan, it's important to create a sustainable, balanced weekly exercise routine that fits seamlessly into your lifestyle. Here's a suggested two-week plan to help you build on your progress and keep the momentum going.

Two-Week Post-Program Plan: Daily Workouts

Day 1

Activity: Cardio + Upper Body Strength

Details: Perform 20 minutes of cardio (e.g., brisk walking, cycling, or jogging) followed by an upper body strength workout. Include exercises such as:

- Chest Press (3 sets of 10-12 reps)
- Bicep Curls (3 sets of 10-12 reps)
- Shoulder Press (3 sets of 10-12 reps)

Day 2

Activity: Flexibility
Details: Dedicate this day to improving flexibility and mobility with yoga, Pilates, or a focused stretching routine. Suggested stretches include:

- Downward Dog
- Seated Forward Fold
- Cat-Cow Pose

Day 3

Activity: Cardio + Lower Body Strength
Details: Start with 20 minutes of cardio, then transition into a lower body workout:

- Squats (3 sets of 10-12 reps)
- Lunges (3 sets of 10-12 reps per leg)
- Leg Press (3 sets of 10-12 reps)

Day 4

Activity: Rest Day

Details: Take a break to allow your body to recover and rejuvenate. Focus on hydration, light walking, and self-care activities.

Day 5

Activity: Cardio + Upper Body Strength

Details: Perform 20 minutes of cardio and follow with an upper-body strength workout:

- Rows (3 sets of 10-12 reps)
- Tricep Extensions (3 sets of 10-12 reps)
- Shoulder Lateral Raises (3 sets of 10-12 reps)

Day 6

Activity: Flexibility

Details: Spend time on gentle yoga, Pilates, or a dedicated stretching session to enhance mobility. Suggested poses include:

- Warrior Pose
- Bridge Pose
- Cobra Stretch

Day 7

Activity: Rest Day

Details: Allow your body and mind a full day of rest. Use this time to reflect on the week's progress and prepare for the next cycle.

Day 8

Activity: Cardio + Lower Body Strength

Details: Start with 20 minutes of cardio, then target your lower body:

- Leg Press (3 sets of 10-12 reps)
- Hamstring Curls (3 sets of 10-12 reps)
- Bulgarian Split Squats (3 sets of 10-12 reps per leg)

Day 9

Activity: Flexibility

Details: Focus on improving your range of motion and relaxing the body with yoga or stretching. Include:

- Child's Pose
- Pigeon Pose
- Side Stretch

Day 10

Activity: Cardio + Upper Body Strength

Details: Perform 20 minutes of cardio, then move into an upper body workout:

- Lat Pulldowns (3 sets of 10-12 reps)
- Chest Flys (3 sets of 10-12 reps)
- Dumbbell Overhead Press (3 sets of 10-12 reps)

Day 11

Activity: Rest Day

Details: Prioritize muscle recovery and mental relaxation. Engage in light activity like walking or meditation, if desired.

Day 12

Activity: Cardio + Lower Body Strength

Details: Combine 20 minutes of cardio with a lower body-focused strength workout:

- Lunges (3 sets of 10-12 reps per leg)
- Calf Raises (3 sets of 10-12 reps)
- Glute Bridges (3 sets of 10-12 reps)

Day 13

Activity: Flexibility

Details: Dedicate time to yoga, Pilates, or a gentle stretching routine. Suggested moves include:

- Standing Forward Bend
- Spinal Twists
- Butterfly Stretch

Day 14

Activity: Rest Day

Details: Complete the week with a full rest day. Reflect on your achievements over the two weeks and prepare for the next phase of your fitness journey.

Additional Tips for the Two-Week Plan:

- Cardio: Any enjoyable activity (e.g., walking, biking, or dancing) is great for building heart health and endurance.
- Strength Training: Alternate between upper and lower body exercises. For beginners, perform two sets, increasing to three sets as you progress.

- Flexibility: Incorporate yoga, Pilates, or focused stretching to support mobility, flexibility, and stress relief.
- Rest Days: Scheduled rest days (4, 7, 11, and 14) allow for recovery and prevent overtraining.

This structured two-week plan offers balance and consistency, building strength, endurance, and flexibility. Modify intensity as needed based on energy and goals, and continue to adjust as your fitness improves. Remember, you don't have to work out all of these days—this is just a sample. If you prefer to split up cardio, strength training, and flexibility on separate days, you can absolutely do that. You have endless options.

Listen to your body and do what works best for you. Just make sure to stay active and aim for at least three days a week of movement that suits your lifestyle and supports your goals.

This exercise bonus is designed to be flexible. It allows you to choose the best options each day while progressing at your own pace.

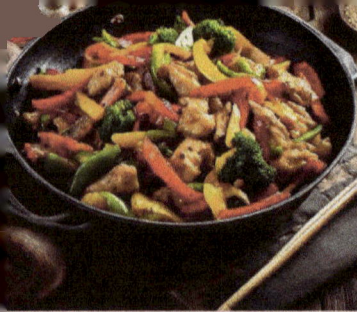

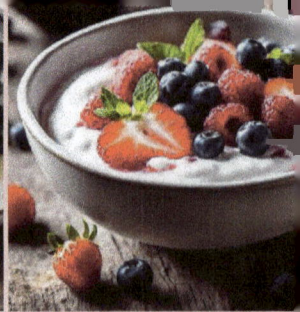

THE
10-DAY RAPID
WEIGHT
LOSS
PLAN

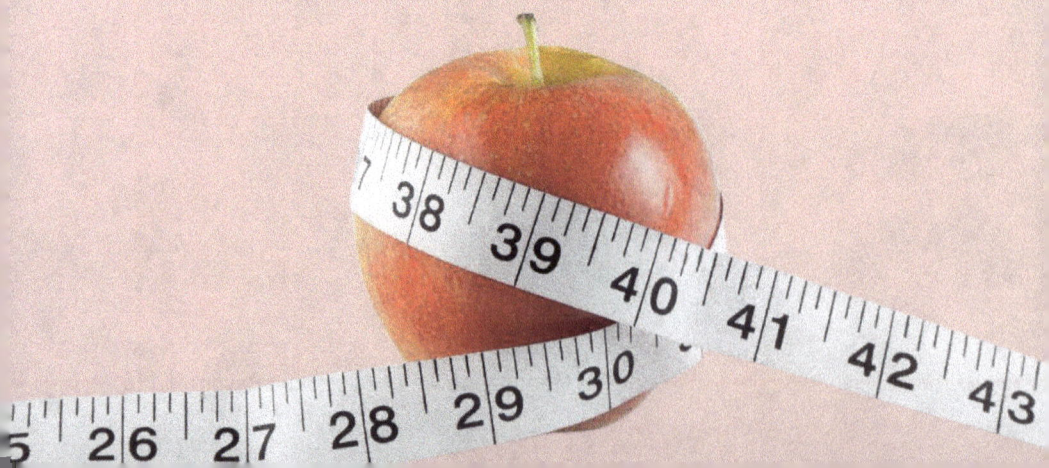

10-DAY

Rapid Weight Loss Plan Menu

Day 1

- Breakfast: Steak and Eggs
- Lunch: Grilled Salmon Salad
- Dinner: Chicken Stir-Fry

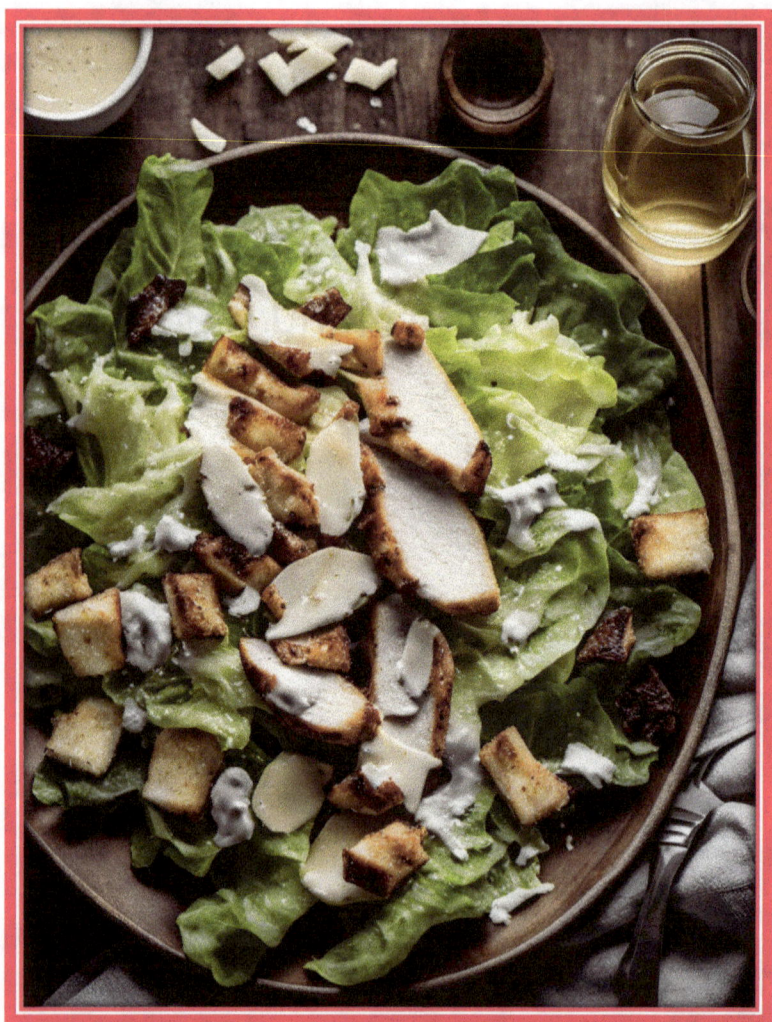

Day 2

- Breakfast: Spinach & Mushroom Omelette
- Lunch: Chicken Caesar Salad
- Dinner: Beef and Vegetable Skewers

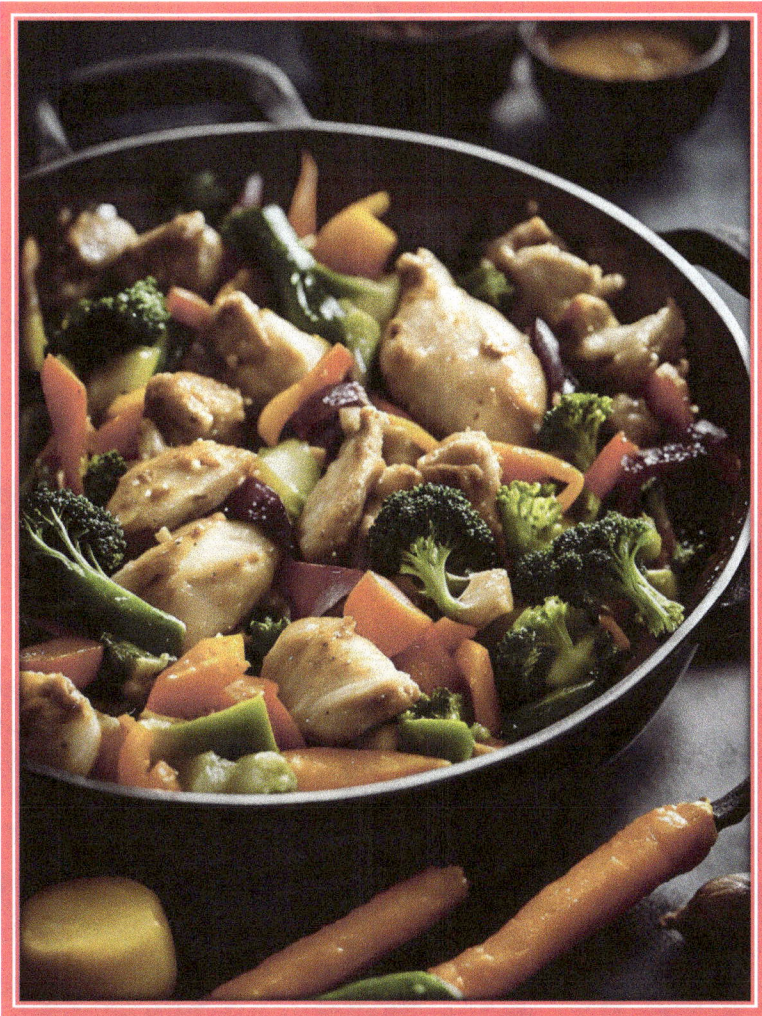

Day 3

- Breakfast: Scrambled Eggs with Smoked Salmon
- Lunch: Turkey Lettuce Wraps
- Dinner: Shrimp & Asparagus Stir-Fry

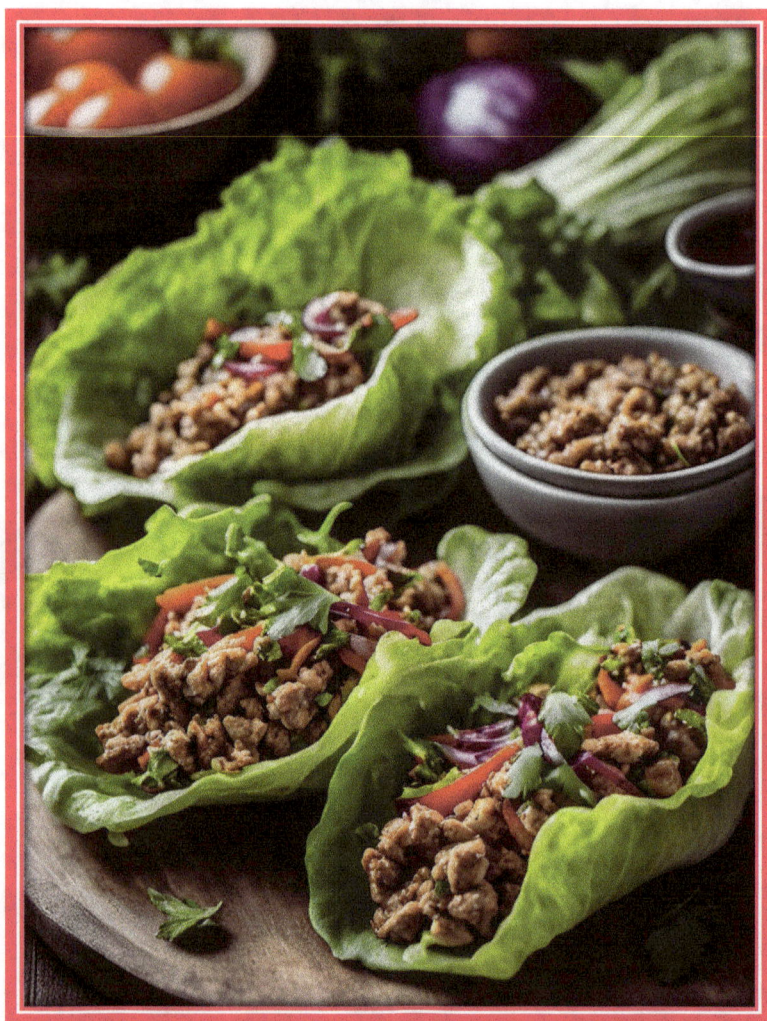

Day 4

- Breakfast: Veggie & Cheese Omelette
- Lunch: Grilled Chicken with Mixed Greens
- Dinner: Beef & Broccoli Stir-Fry

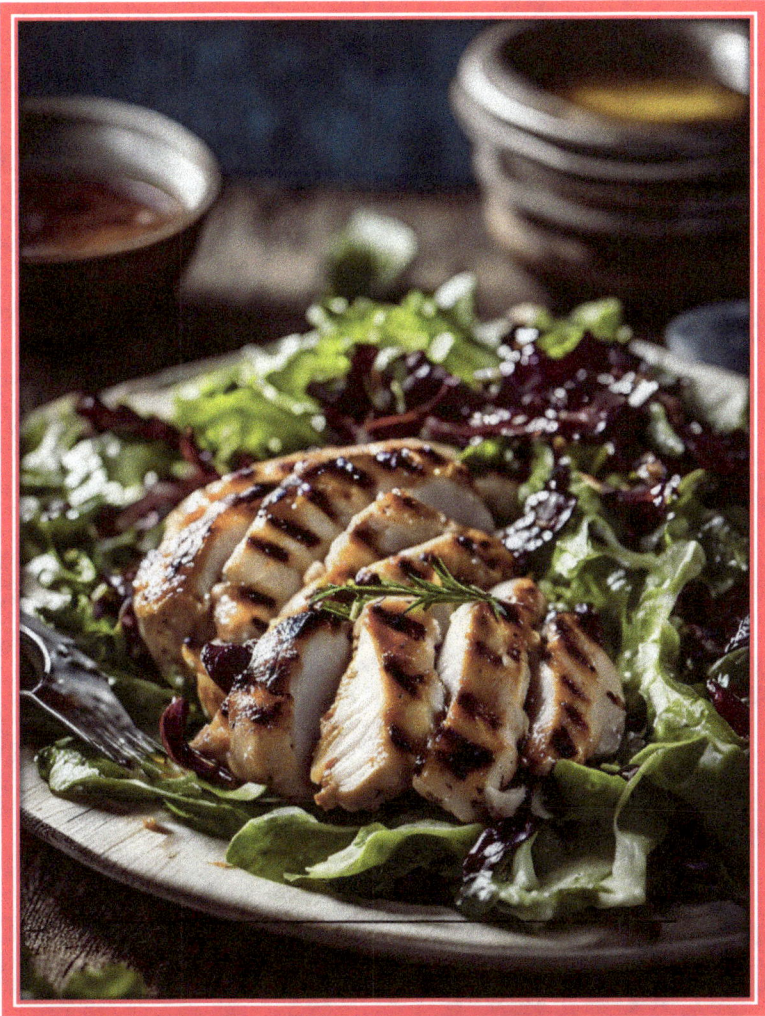

Day 5

- Breakfast: Greek Yogurt Bowl
- Lunch: Tuna Salad Lettuce Wraps
- Dinner: Baked Salmon with Asparagus

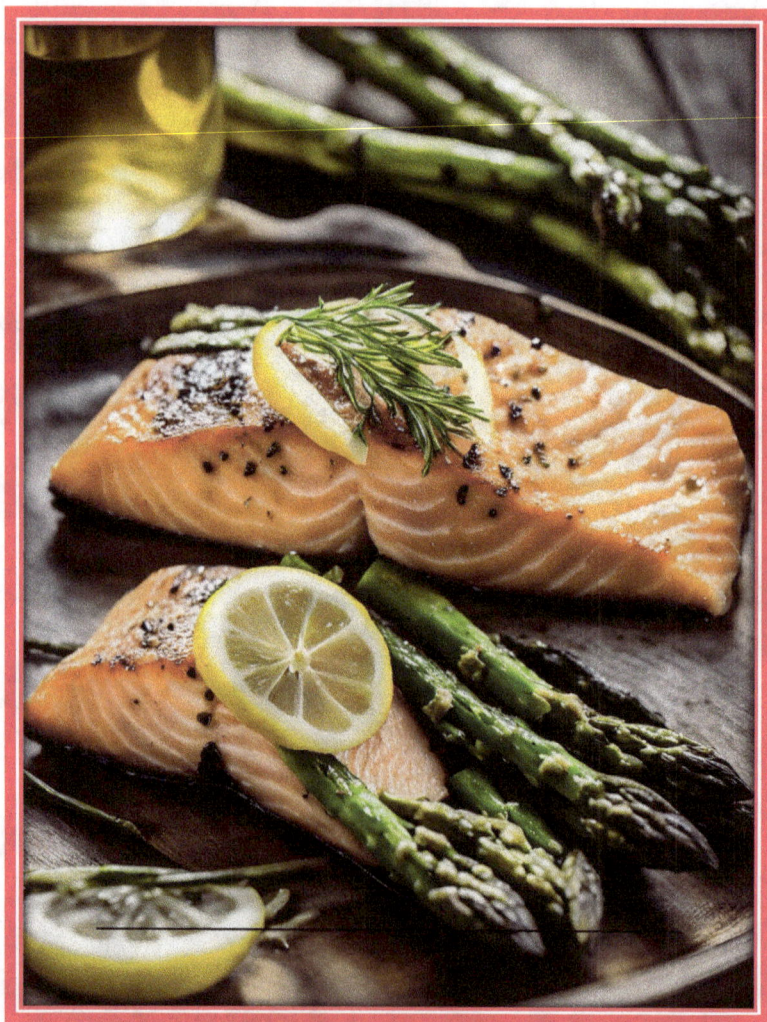

Day 6

- Breakfast: Avocado & Egg Plate
- Lunch: Beef & Zucchini Stir-Fry
- Dinner: Lemon Garlic Shrimp

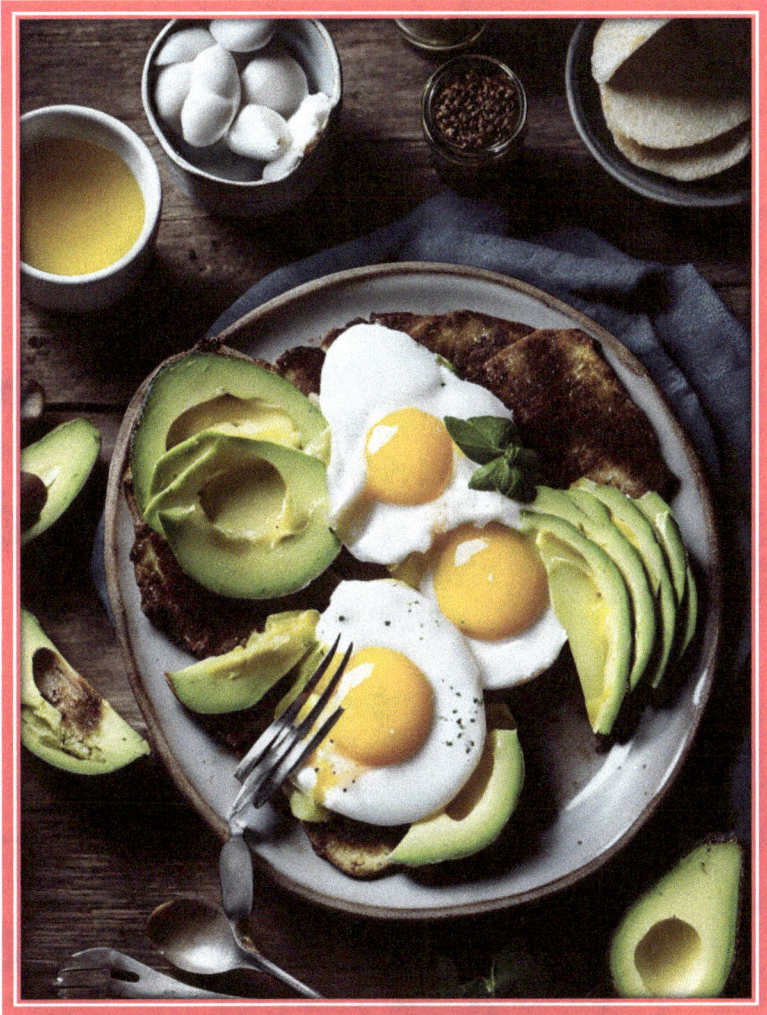

Day 7

- Breakfast: Steak & Eggs
- Lunch: Chicken Caesar Salad
- Dinner: Baked Cod with Steamed Spinach

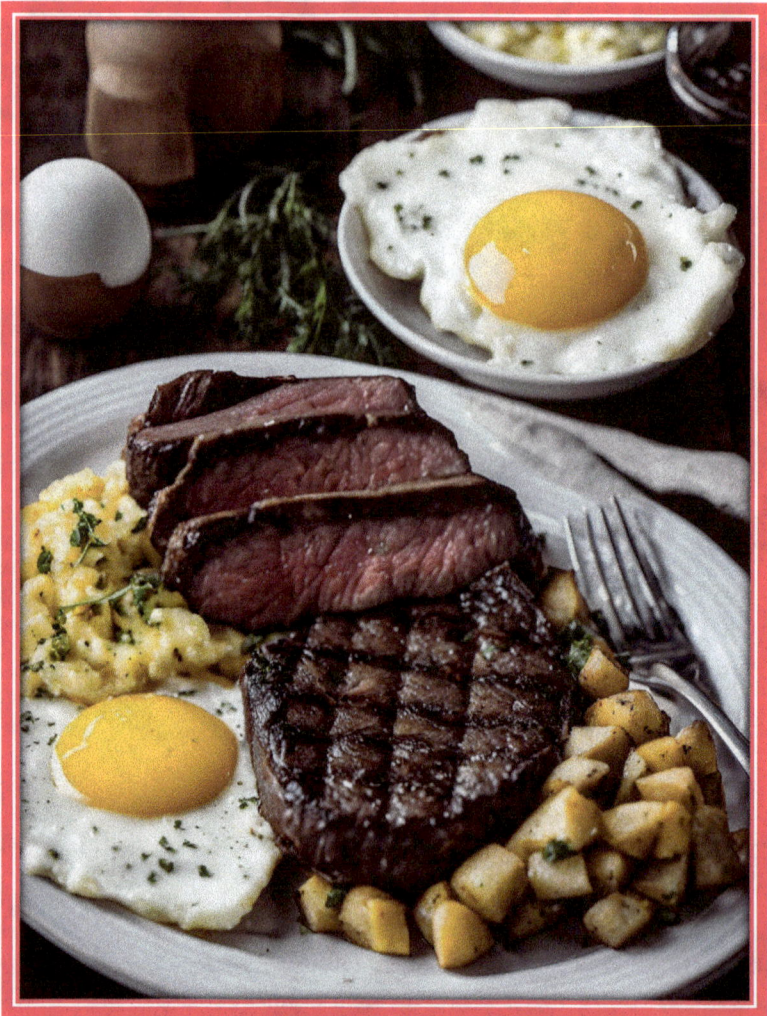

Day 8

- Breakfast: Veggie Omelette with Spinach & Mushrooms
- Lunch: Shrimp & Avocado Salad
- Dinner: Grilled Salmon & Steamed Asparagus

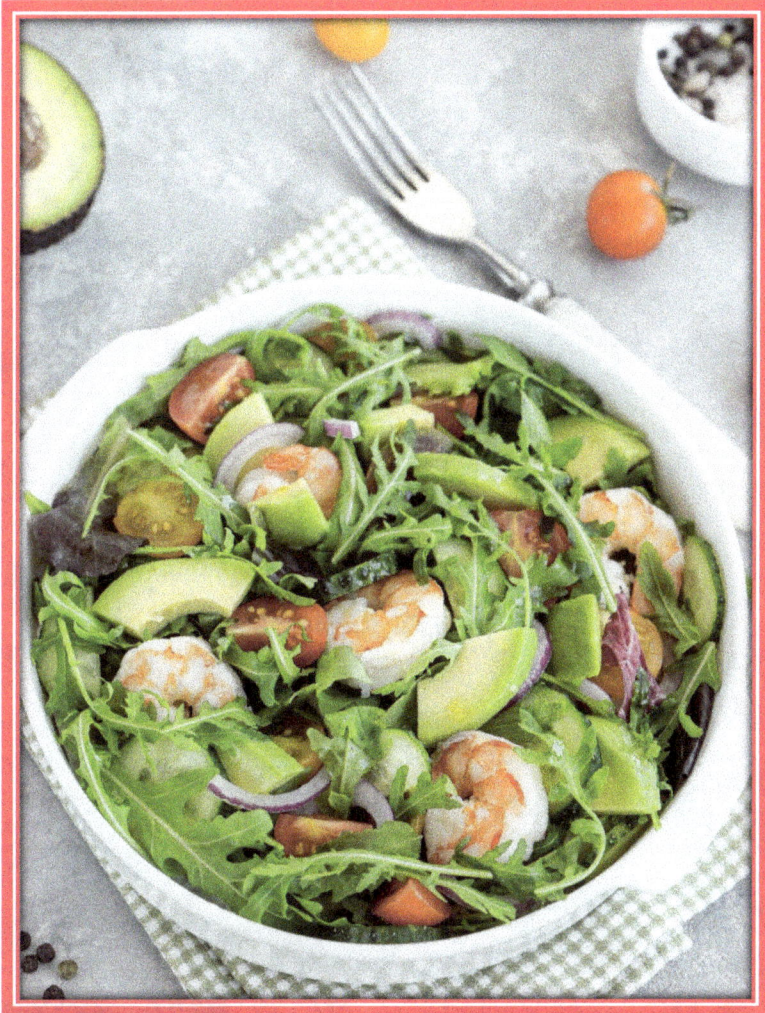

Day 9

- Breakfast: Greek Yogurt with Berries
- Lunch: Chicken & Bell Pepper Stir-Fry
- Dinner: Tilapia with Green Beans

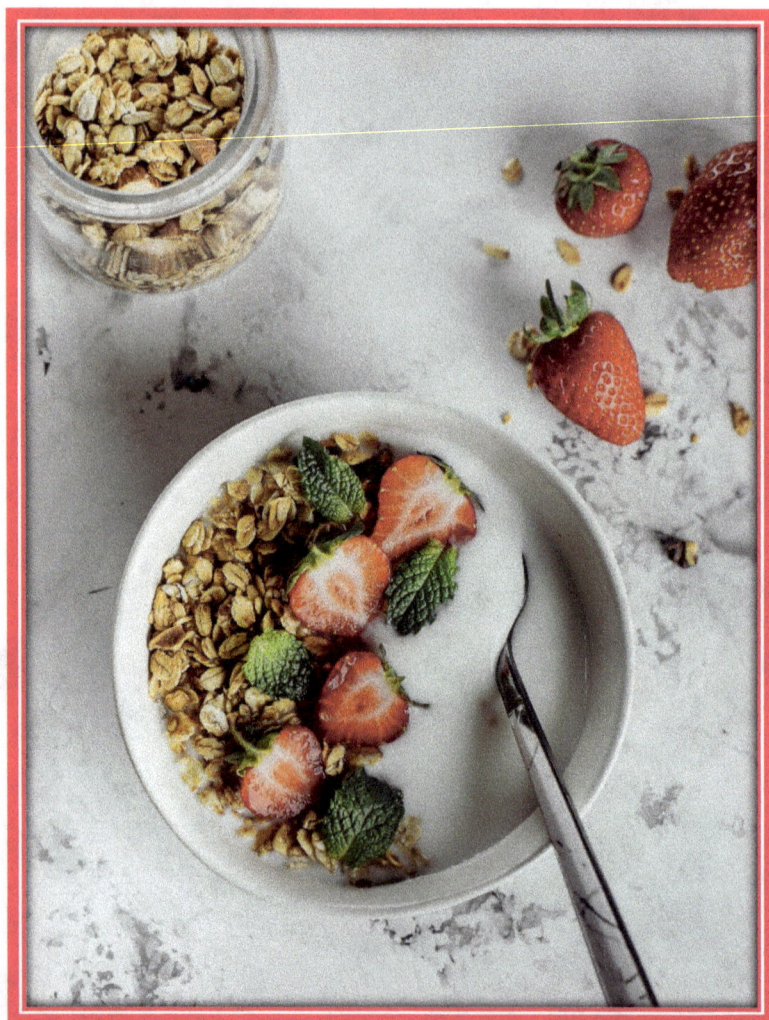

Day 10

- Breakfast: Scrambled Eggs with Turkey Sausage
- Lunch: Tuna Salad on Mixed Greens
- Dinner: Baked Chicken Thighs with Broccoli

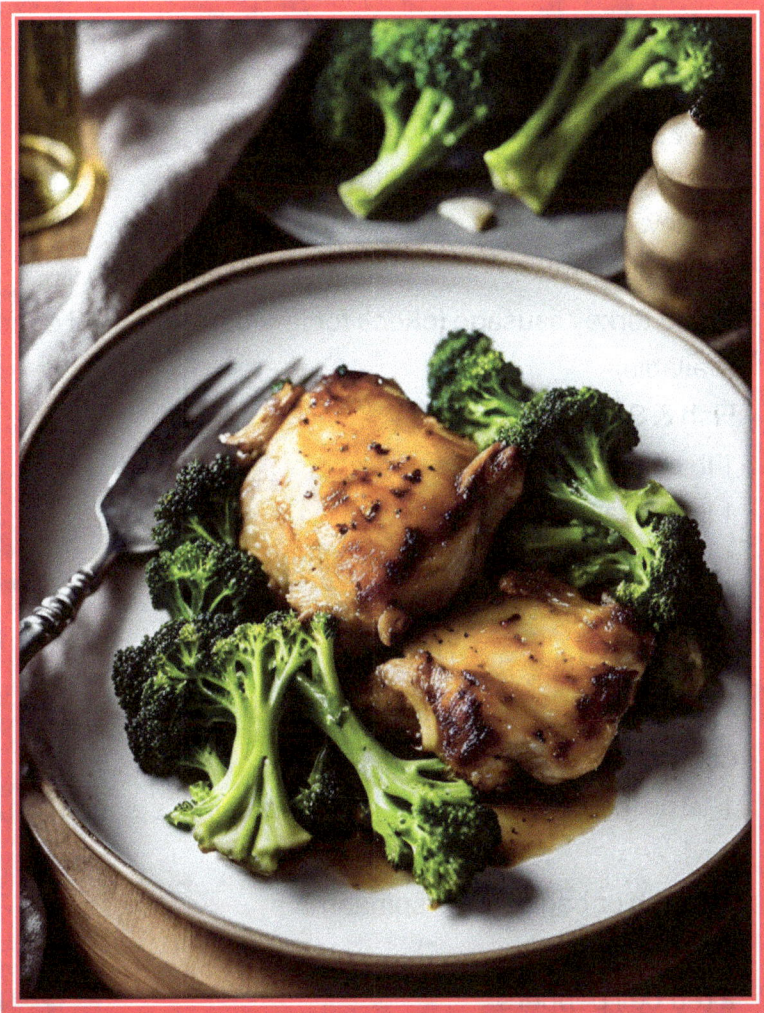

10-Day Rapid Weight-Loss Plan Grocery List

Proteins

- Eggs: 2 dozen large eggs
- Chicken:
- 2 lbs boneless, skinless chicken breast
- 1 lb chicken thighs (bone-in or boneless)
- Beef:
- 2 lbs ground beef (90% lean or higher)
- 1 lb steak (such as sirloin or ribeye)
- Turkey:
- 1 lb ground turkey
- 1/2 lb turkey sausage (check for low-carb, uncured options if available)
- Fish & Seafood:
- 1 lb salmon filets
- 1 lb tilapia filets
- 1/2 lb shrimp, peeled and deveined
- 2 cans tuna in water (about 5 oz each)

Vegetables

- Leafy Greens:
- 1 large bag of mixed greens (or romaine, spinach, arugula mix)
- 1 bunch or bag of fresh spinach
- Other Vegetables:
- 2 red bell peppers

- 2 green bell peppers
- 1 large cucumber
- 1 lb broccoli
- 1 bunch asparagus
- 1 lb green beans
- 1 small head cauliflower
- 1 small head of lettuce (optional for additional salads)

Fruits

- Berries:
- Strawberries (1 pint)
- Raspberries (1 pint)
- Blueberries (1 pint)

Healthy Fats

- Avocado: 2 avocados
- Olive Oil: 1 bottle (extra virgin preferred)
- Butter or Ghee: 1 small tub or stick (grass-fed if available)
- Feta Cheese (1 small container)
- Parmesan Cheese (1 small container)

Pantry Items & Seasonings

- Herbs & Seasonings:
- Salt (Himalayan, Redmond, or sea salt recommended)
- Black pepper
- Garlic powder
- Lemon zest or fresh lemon
- Other:

- 1 small bottle of olive oil-based or high-fat dressing (optional for salads)
- Garlic Cloves (4 cloves or 1 bulb)
- Soy Sauce or Coconut Aminos (small bottle)
- Balsamic Vinegar (small bottle)
- Lemon (1-2 for juice and garnish)

Optional/Recommended Supplements

- Electrolyte Powder or You can always use Himalayan, Redmond, or sea salt

Rapid Weight-Loss Approved Foods List

Proteins

- Beef (various cuts, grass-fed preferred)
- Chicken (breast, thighs, drumsticks, pasture-raised preferred)
- Turkey (bacon, ground or whole cuts)
- Fish (wild-caught salmon, tilapia, cod)
- Shrimp
- Eggs (whole eggs)
- Bacon
- Smoked salmon
- Grass-fed beef protein powder
- Egg white protein powder

Fats

- Olive oil
- Coconut oil
- Butter (grass-fed preferred)
- Avocado oil
- Full-fat sour cream
- Full-fat cheeses (Feta, Parmesan etc)
- Heavy cream
- Coconut milk
- Almond milk
- Dressings:
- Balsamic dressing
- Full-fat Caesar dressing
- Full-fat ranch dressing

Fruits

- Avocado
- Strawberries
- Raspberries
- Blueberries
- Lemon (for flavoring)

Vegetables (Low-Glycemic)

- Spinach
- Kale
- Mixed greens
- Asparagus
- Zucchini
- Broccoli
- Cauliflower
- Bell peppers
- Brussels sprouts
- Cucumber
- Green beans
- Cherry tomatoes

Beverages

- Water
- Tea (green, black, herbal)
- Coffee (plain, can add approved creamers or sweeteners)

Spices, Seasonings, and Condiments

- Sea salt
- Himalayan salt
- Redmond salt
- Black pepper
- Onion powder
- Garlic powder
- Lemon juice
- Fresh herbs (parsley, dill, etc.)
- Apple cider vinegar
- Stevia (natural, no additives)
- Monk fruit sweetener (natural, no additives)

Optional/Recommended Supplements

- Electrolyte Powder or You can always use Himalayan, Redmond, or sea salt

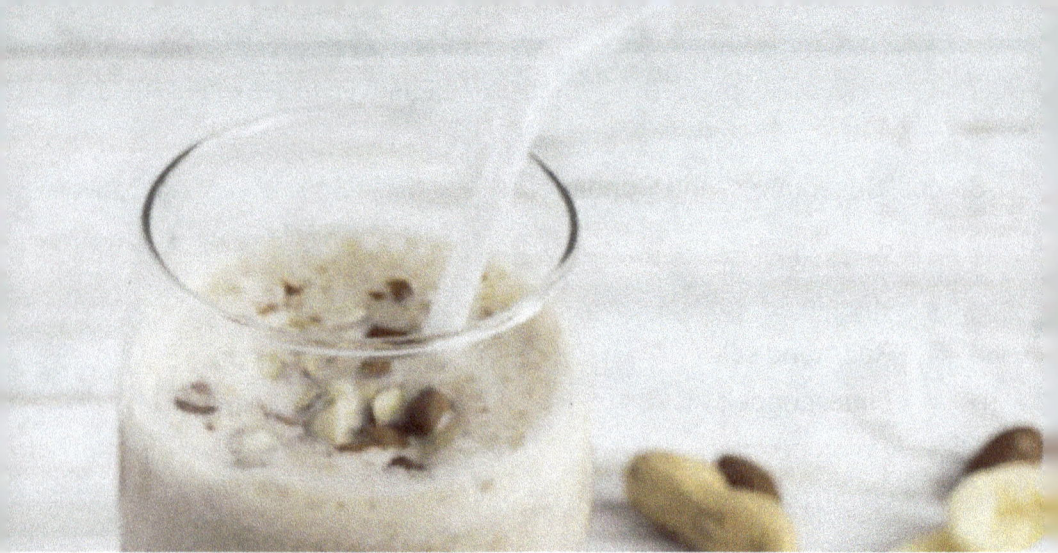

SMOOTHIE RECIPES

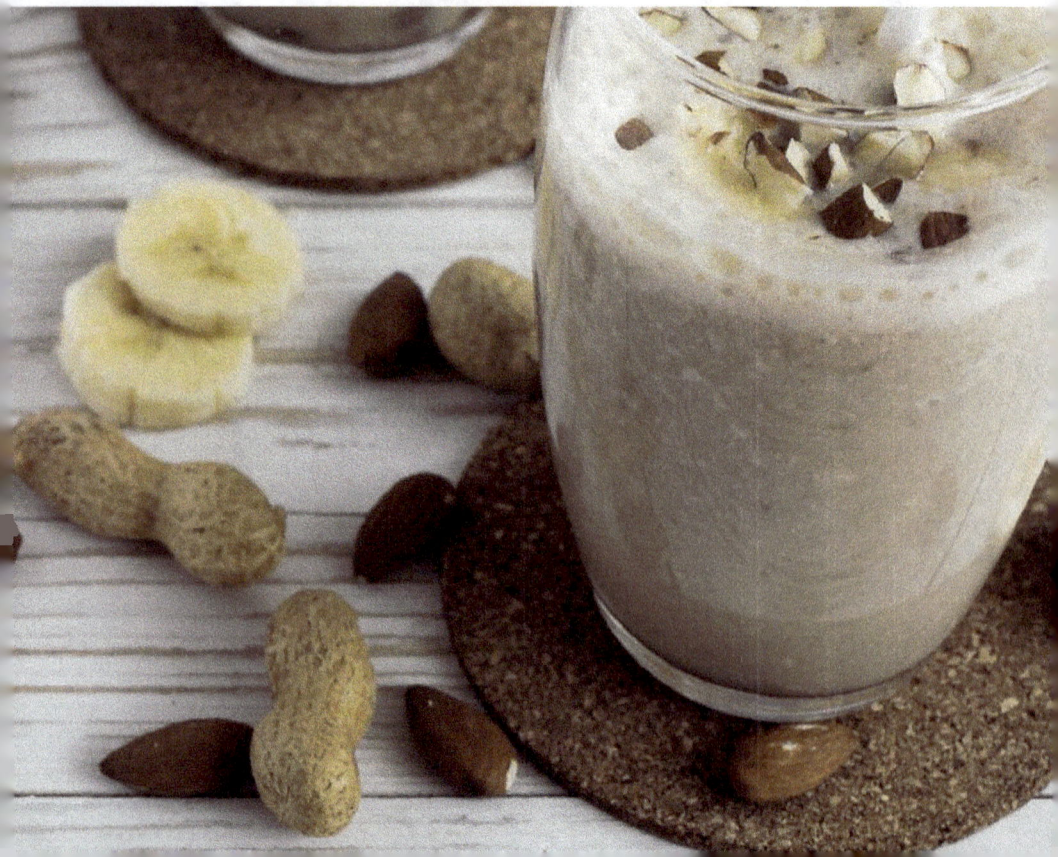

Grass-Fed Beef Protein Smoothie

INGREDIENTS:

- 1 scoop grass-fed beef protein powder
- 8 - 12 oz of unsweetened
- almond milk, coconut milk or water
- 1/2 cup berries (blueberries, raspberries, or strawberries)
- 1/2 avocado (optional for creaminess)
- 1-2 ice cubes

INSTRUCTIONS:

1. Place all ingredients in a blender and blend until smooth.
2. Adjust consistency by adding more liquid if needed.
3. Enjoy immediately.

Egg White Protein Smoothie

INGREDIENTS:

- 1 scoop egg white protein powder
- 8 - 12 oz if unsweetened almond milk, coconut milk or water
- 1/2 cup berries (blueberries, raspberries, or strawberries)
- 1-2 ice cubes

INSTRUCTIONS:

1. Combine all ingredients in a blender and blend until smooth.
2. Add more liquid if a thinner consistency is desired.
3. Drink right away for optimal freshness.

Day 1 Reminder

Hydration: Drink at least half your body weight in ounces of water daily. For added electrolytes, add a pinch of Himalayan or sea salt to your water.

Protein Focus: Aim for at least 30g of protein per meal to support lean muscle and satiety.

Positive Mindset: Repeat today's mantra, "I am beautiful, I am strong, and I deserve to be happy." Set a positive intention for the day.

Breakfast: Steak and Eggs

INGREDIENTS:

- 5 oz grass-fed beef steak
- 2 large eggs
- Salt and pepper to taste

INSTRUCTIONS:

1. Season the steak with salt and pepper.
2. Heat a skillet over medium-high heat. Add the steak and cook for 3-4 minutes per side, or until it reaches your preferred level of doneness.
3. Remove steak from the skillet and let it rest for a minute.
4. In the same skillet, crack the eggs and cook sunny side up or scramble as desired.

5. Serve the steak with the eggs on the side.

NUTRITION FACTS:

- Calories: 400, Protein: 35g, Carbs: 0g, Fat: 28g

Lunch: Grilled Salmon Salad

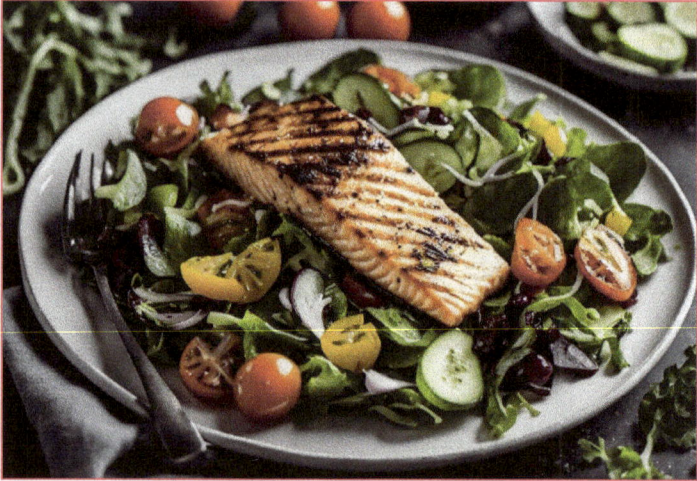

INGREDIENTS:

- 5 oz salmon filet
- 2 cups mixed greens
- 1/2 cucumber, sliced
- 5 cherry tomatoes, halved
- 1 tbsp olive oil
- 1 tsp lemon juice
- Salt and pepper to taste

INSTRUCTIONS:

1. Preheat the grill or use a skillet over medium heat. Season the salmon with salt and pepper.
2. Grill or cook the salmon for 4-5 minutes per side, until it flakes easily with a fork.

3. Arrange mixed greens, cucumber, and cherry tomatoes on a plate.
4. Top the salad with the grilled salmon, drizzle with olive oil and lemon juice, and serve.

NUTRITION FACTS:

- Calories: 450, Protein: 40g, Carbs: 10g, Fat: 28g

Dinner: Chicken Stir-Fry

INGREDIENTS:

- 5 oz chicken breast, sliced
- 1 cup bell peppers, sliced
- 1/2 cup broccoli florets
- 1 tbsp coconut oil
- 1 tbsp soy sauce

INSTRUCTIONS:

1. Heat coconut oil in a skillet over medium heat.
2. Add the chicken slices to the skillet and cook until browned, about 5 minutes.
3. Add bell peppers and broccoli to the skillet and stir-fry until vegetables are tender, about 3-4 minutes.
4. Add soy sauce, stir well, and serve hot.

TOTAL NUTRITION FOR DAY 1:

- Calories: 1230 Protein: 107g Carbs: 18g Fat: 78g

NUTRITION FACTS:

- Calories: 380, Protein: 32g, Carbs: 8g, Fat: 22g

Day 2 Reminder

Hydration: Continue to drink water throughout the day and consider herbal teas for variety.

Mindful Eating: Take time to enjoy each meal without distractions. This helps with digestion and satisfaction.

Today's Mantra: "I am in control of my choices, and each choice brings me closer to my goals."

Breakfast: Spinach & Mushroom Omelette

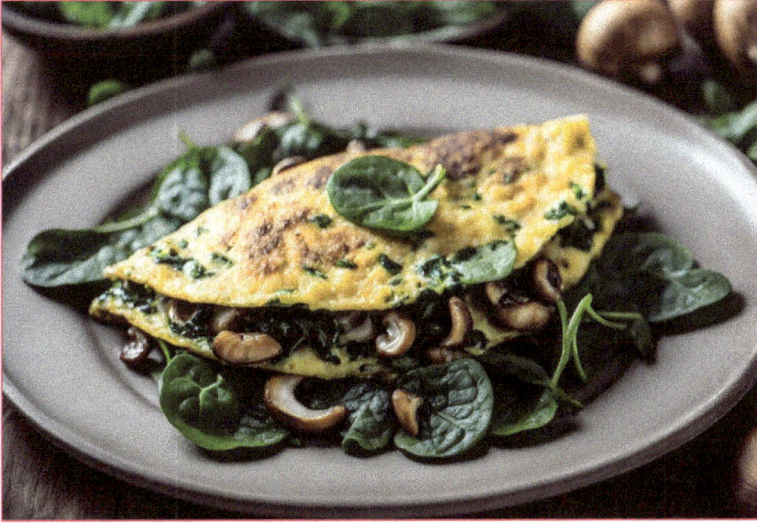

INGREDIENTS:

- 3 large eggs
- 1/2 cup fresh spinach
- 1/4 cup sliced mushrooms
- 1 tbsp olive oil or butter
- Salt and pepper to taste

INSTRUCTIONS:

- Heat olive oil or butter in a skillet over medium heat.
- Add mushrooms and spinach, sautéing until soft (about 2-3 minutes).

- In a bowl, whisk the eggs with a pinch of salt and pepper, then pour into the skilled.
- Cook until eggs are set, fold the omelet in half, and serve warm.

NUTRITION FACTS:

- Calories: 320, Protein: 24g, Carbs: 5g, Fat: 24g

Lunch: Chicken Caesar Salad

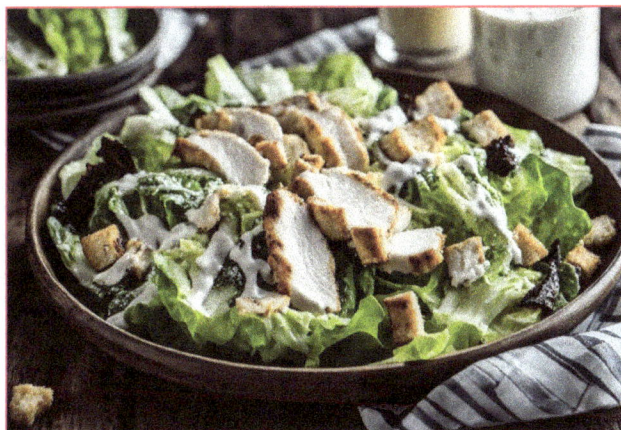

INGREDIENTS:

- 5 oz grilled chicken breast, sliced
- 2 cups romaine lettuce, chopped
- 1 tbsp Caesar dressing
- 1 tbsp grated Parmesan cheese (optional)
- Salt and pepper to taste

INSTRUCTIONS:

1. Place chopped romaine on a plate. Add grilled chicken slices on top of the lettuce.
2. Drizzle with Caesar dressing and sprinkle with Parmesan, if using. Season with a little salt and pepper to taste.

NUTRITION FACTS:

- Calories: 400, Protein: 35g, Carbs: 7g, Fat: 26g

Dinner: Beef and Vegetable Skewers

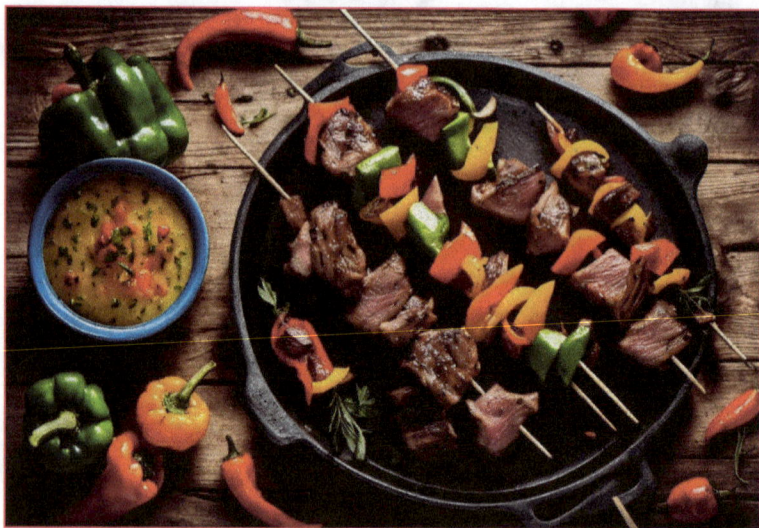

INGREDIENTS:

- 5 oz beef sirloin, cut into 1-inch cubes
- 1/2 cup bell peppers, cut into squares
- 1/2 cup zucchini, sliced
- 1 tbsp olive oil
- Salt, pepper, and garlic powder to taste

INSTRUCTIONS:

1. Preheat grill or oven broiler to medium-high heat.
2. Thread beef, bell peppers, and zucchini onto skewers, alternating ingredients.
3. Brush with olive oil and season with salt, pepper, and garlic powder.

4. Grill or broil for about 8-10 minutes, turning occasionally, until beef is cooked to your liking and veggies are tender.

TOTAL NUTRITION FOR DAY 2:

- Calories: 1200 Protein: 97g Carbs: 18g Fat: 84g

NUTRITION FACTS:

- Calories: 48, Protein: 38g, Carbs: 6g, Fat: 34g

Day 3 Reminder

Hydration & Electrolytes: Continue to drink water and add a pinch of Himalayan or sea salt to one of your water servings today to replenish electrolytes.

Mindset for Success: Reflect on how far you've come, even in these few days, and acknowledge your commitment.

Today's Mantra: "I am dedicated to my health and wellness journey, and each step I take brings me closer to my goals."

Breakfast: Scrambled Eggs with Smoked Salmon

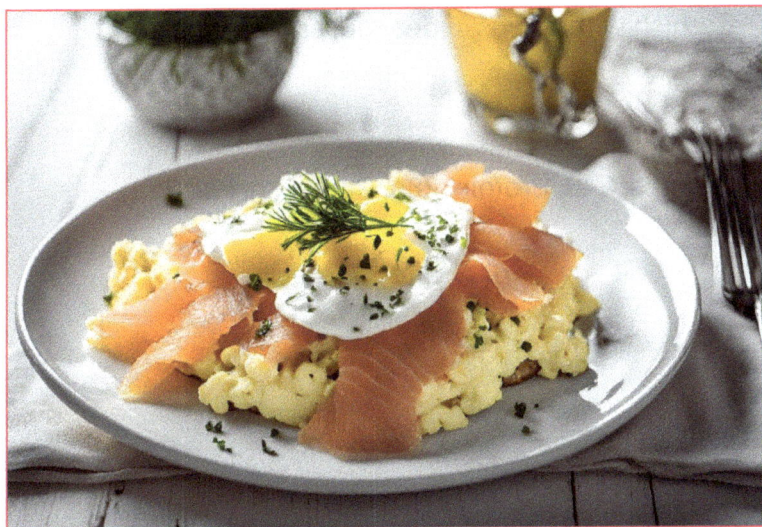

INGREDIENTS:

- 3 large eggs
- 2 oz smoked salmon, chopped
- 1 tbsp chives, chopped (optional)
- 1 tbsp butter or olive oil
- Salt and pepper to taste

INSTRUCTIONS:

1. Heat butter or olive oil in a skillet over medium heat.
2. Crack the eggs into a bowl, whisk them, and season with a pinch of salt and pepper.

3. Pour eggs into the skillet and cook, stirring gently, until they begin to set.
4. Add chopped smoked salmon and continue cooking until eggs are fully scrambled.
5. Garnish with chives, if desired, and serve warm.

NUTRITION FACTS:

- Calories: 340, Protein: 28g, Carbs: 3g, Fat: 25g

Lunch: Turkey Lettuce Wraps

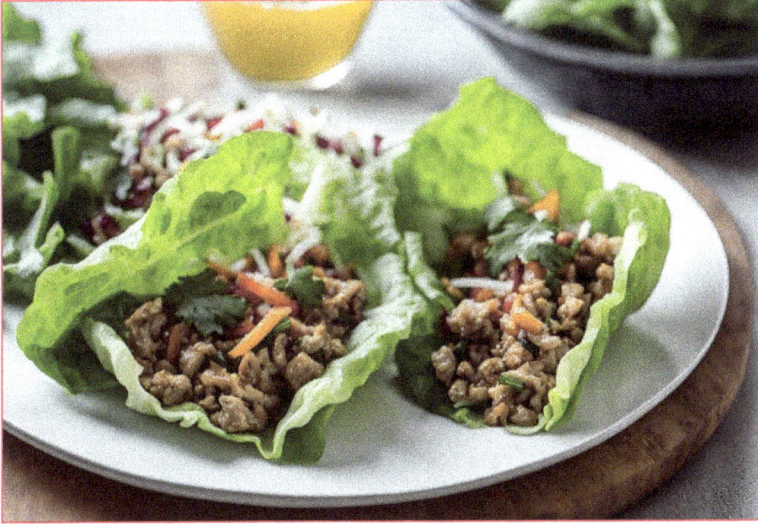

INGREDIENTS:

- 5 oz ground turkey
- 1/4 cup bell peppers, diced
- 1/4 cup onion, diced
- 1 tbsp olive oil
- Salt, pepper, and garlic powder to taste
- 4 large lettuce leaves for wrapping

INSTRUCTIONS:

1. Heat olive oil in a skillet over medium heat. Add ground turkey, bell peppers, and onion to the skillet. Cook until turkey is browned and vegetables are soft (about 8-10 minutes).

2. Season with salt, pepper, and garlic powder. Spoon turkey mixture onto lettuce leaves, wrap, and enjoy as a wrap or taco-style meal.

NUTRITION FACTS:

- Calories: 350, Protein: 32g, Carbs: 6g, Fat: 22g

Dinner: Shrimp & Asparagus Stir-Fry

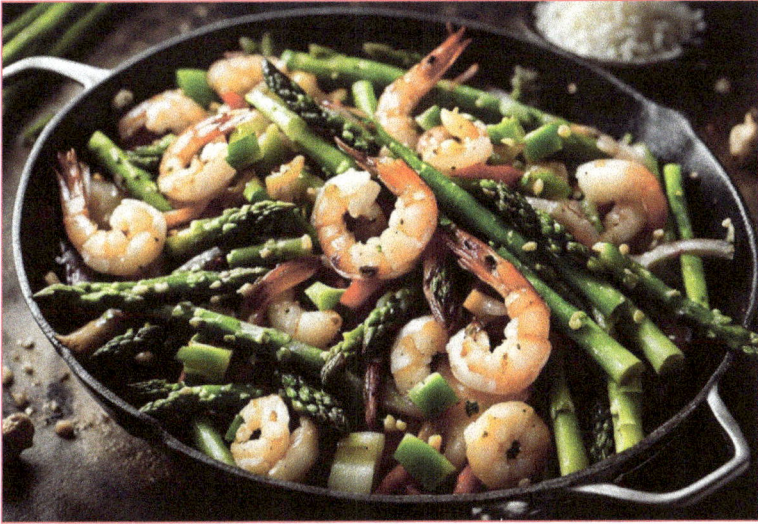

INGREDIENTS:

- 5 oz shrimp, peeled and deveined
- 1 cup asparagus, trimmed and cut into pieces
- 1 tbsp coconut oil or olive oil
- 1 tbsp lemon juice
- Salt, pepper, and garlic powder to taste

INSTRUCTIONS:

- Heat oil in a skillet over medium-high heat.
- Add shrimp and asparagus to the skillet and cook for 5-7 minutes, until shrimp is pink and asparagus is tender.

- Season with salt, pepper, and garlic powder, then drizzle with lemon juice before serving.

TOTAL NUTRITION FOR DAY 3:

- Calories: 1000 Protein: 95g Carbs: 16g Fat: 65g

NUTRITION FACTS:

- Calories: 310, Protein: 35g, Carbs: 7g, Fat: 18g

Day 4 Reminder

Hydration & Electrolytes: Remember to keep your water intake up and add electrolytes as needed. Adding a slice of lemon or lime to your water can make it more enjoyable.

Gratitude Practice: Reflect on three things you're grateful for today.

Today's Mantra: "I am worthy of good health and lasting change."

Breakfast: Veggie & Cheese Omelette

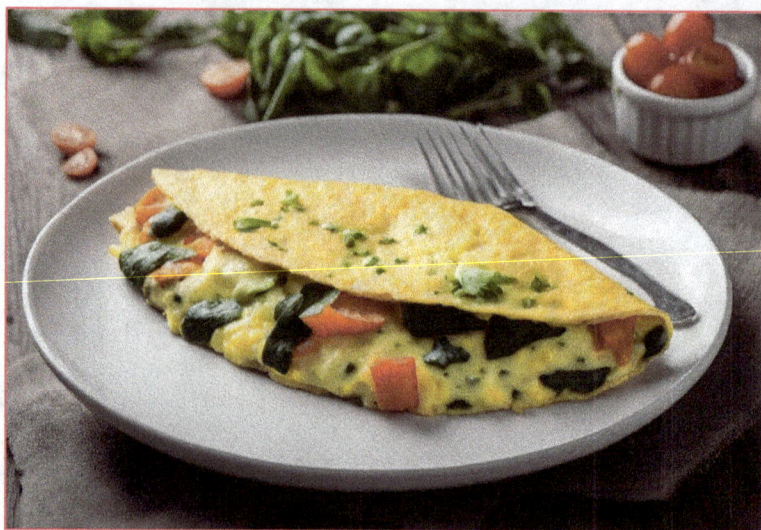

INGREDIENTS:

- 3 large eggs
- 1/4 cup bell peppers, diced
- 1/4 cup spinach
- 1 tbsp shredded cheese (optional)
- 1 tbsp olive oil or butter
- Salt and pepper to taste

INSTRUCTIONS:

- Heat olive oil or butter in a skillet over medium heat.
- Add bell peppers and spinach, sautéing until tender.

- Whisk eggs in a bowl, season with salt and pepper, then pour into the skillet.
- Cook until eggs are set, folding in half and adding cheese if desired. Serve warm.

NUTRITION FACTS:

- Calories: 320, Protein: 24g, Carbs: 5g, Fat: 24g

Lunch: Grilled Chicken with Mixed Greens

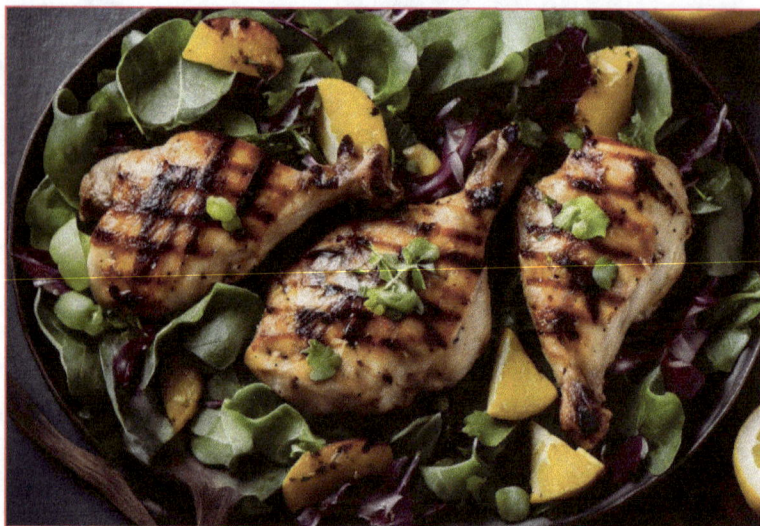

INGREDIENTS:

- 5 oz grilled chicken breast
- 2 cups mixed greens
- 1/4 cucumber, sliced
- 5 cherry tomatoes, halved
- 1 tbsp olive oil
- 1 tsp balsamic vinegar
- Salt and pepper to taste

INSTRUCTIONS:

- Arrange mixed greens, cucumber, and cherry tomatoes on a plate.

- Top with grilled chicken slices, drizzle with olive oil and balsamic vinegar, and season with salt and pepper.

NUTRITION FACTS:

- Calories: 400, Protein: 35g, Carbs: 8g, Fat: 26g

Dinner: Beef & Broccoli Stir-Fry

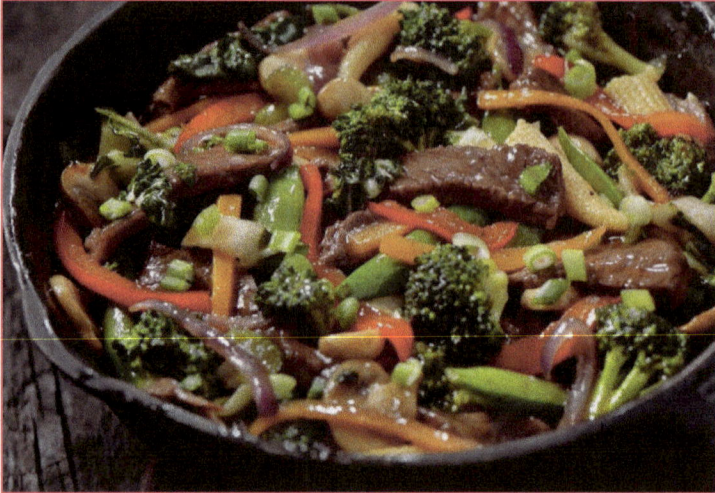

INGREDIENTS:

- 5 oz beef sirloin, thinly sliced
- 1 cup broccoli florets
- 1 tbsp coconut oil
- 1 tbsp soy sauce
- Salt and pepper to taste

INSTRUCTIONS:

- Heat coconut oil in a skillet over medium- high heat.
- Add beef slices and cook until browned, about 4 minutes.
- Add broccoli and stir-fry for another 3-4 minutes, until tender.
- Drizzle with soy sauce, season with salt and pepper, and serve.

TOTAL NUTRITION FOR DAY 4:

- Calories: 1140 Protein: 94g Carbs: 20g Fat: 78g

NUTRITION FACTS:

- Calories: 420, Protein: 35g, Carbs: 7g, Fat: 28g

Day 5 Reminder

Hydration & Movement: Aim to move throughout the day. A quick walk or light stretching can help boost your mood and energy levels.

Reflect on Progress: Take a moment to think about how you feel compared to Day 1.

Today's Mantra: "Every small step is progress, and I am proud of each one."

Breakfast: Greek Yogurt Bowl

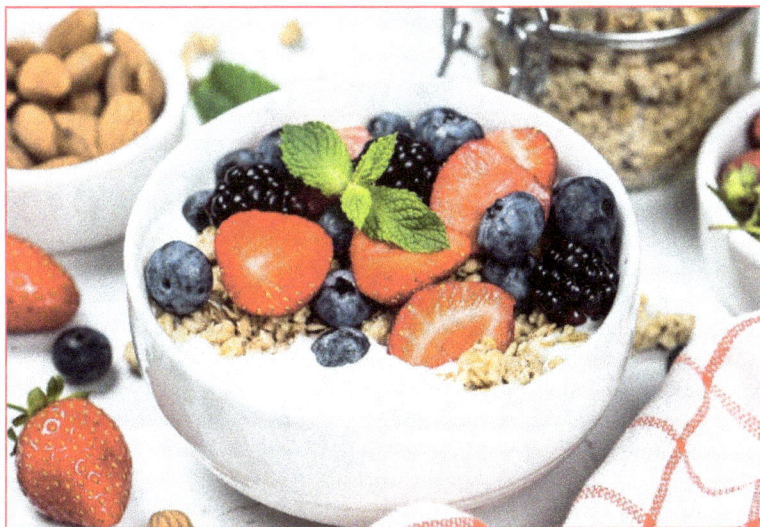

INGREDIENTS:

- 3/4 cup unsweetened Greek yogurt
- 1/4 cup fresh berries (such as strawberries or blueberries)

INSTRUCTIONS:

1. Place Greek yogurt in a bowl.
2. Top with berries. Enjoy immediately.

NUTRITION FACTS:

- Calories: 200, Protein: 18g, Carbs: 10g,Fat: 8g

Lunch: Tuna Salad Lettuce Wraps

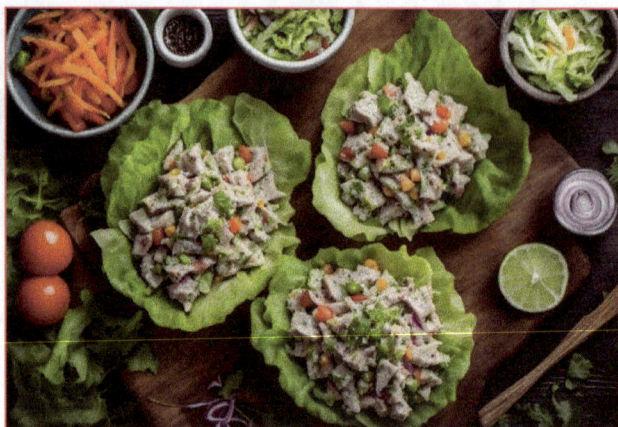

INGREDIENTS:

- 5 oz canned tuna, drained
- 2 tbsp mayonnaise
- 1 tbsp diced celery
- 1 tbsp diced onion
- Salt and pepper to taste
- 4 large lettuce leaves

INSTRUCTIONS:

1. In a bowl, mix tuna, mayonnaise, celery, and onion.
2. Season with salt and pepper.
3. Spoon mixture into lettuce leaves, wrap, and enjoy

NUTRITION FACTS:

- Calories: 350, Protein: 32g, Carbs: 5g, Fat: 24g

Dinner: Baked Salmon with Asparagus

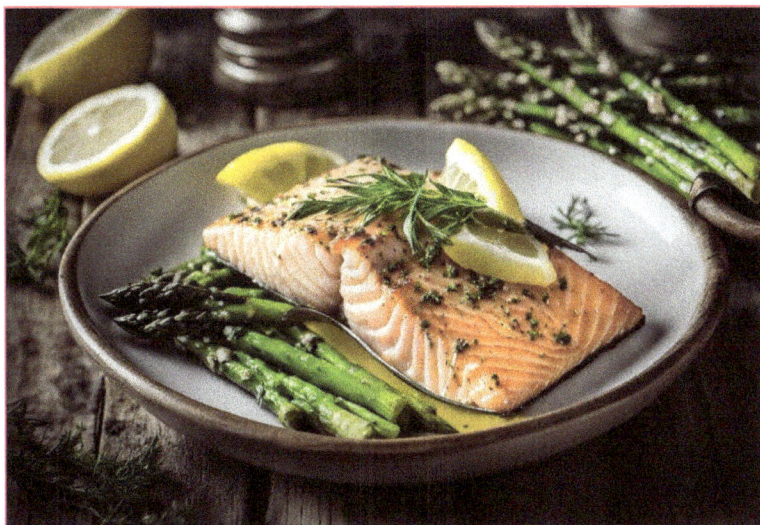

INGREDIENTS:

- 5 oz salmon filet
- 1 cup asparagus spears
- 1 tbsp olive oil
- Salt, pepper, and garlic powder to taste

INSTRUCTIONS:

1. Preheat the oven to 400°F (200°C).
2. Place salmon and asparagus on a baking sheet, drizzle with olive oil, and season with salt, pepper, and garlic powder.
3. Bake for 12-15 minutes, or until salmon is cooked through and asparagus is tender.

TOTAL NUTRITION FOR DAY 5:

- Calories: 960 Protein: 86g Carbs: 21g Fat: 60g

NUTRITION FACTS:

- Calories: 410, Protein: 36g, Carbs: 6g, Fat: 28g

Day 6 Reminder

Hydration & Self-Care: Keep up with hydration, and try to schedule a few minutes for self-care today—whether it's a short walk, meditating, or enjoying a moment of quiet.

Stay Consistent: Consistency brings results, so celebrate each day you stick to your plan.

Today's Mantra: "I am committed to my health and my happiness."

Breakfast: Avocado & Egg Plate

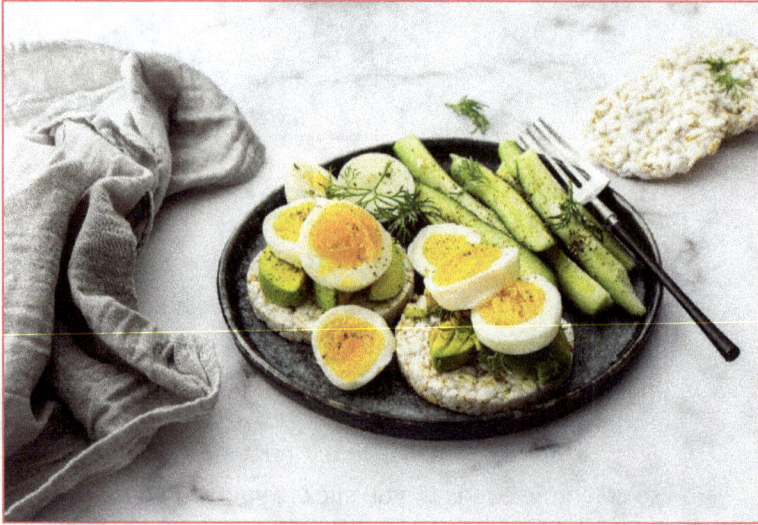

INGREDIENTS:

- 2 large eggs
- 1/2 avocado, sliced
- Salt, pepper, and paprika to taste

INSTRUCTIONS:

1. Soft-boil or hard-boil the eggs as desired. Slice the avocado and place it on a plate alongside the eggs.
2. Season with salt, pepper, and a sprinkle of paprika for added flavor.

NUTRITION FACTS:

- Calories: 300, Protein: 15g, Carbs: 6g, Fat: 24g

Lunch: Beef & Zucchini Stir-Fry

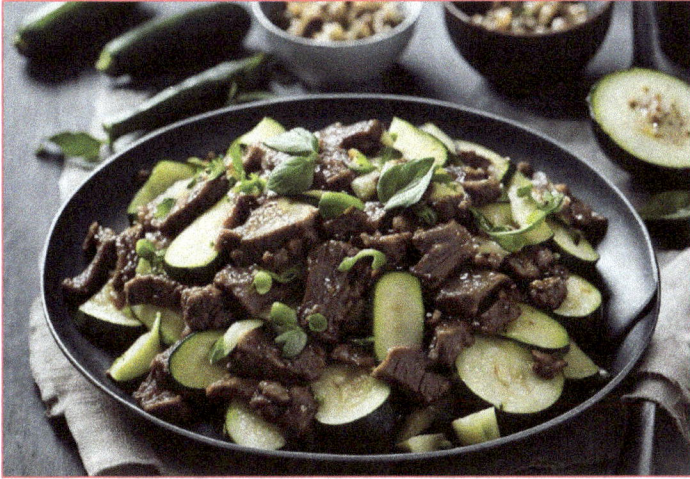

INGREDIENTS:

- 5 oz ground beef (grass-fed if possible)
- 1 cup zucchini, sliced
- 1 tbsp olive oil
- Salt, pepper, and garlic powder to taste

INSTRUCTIONS:

1. Heat olive oil in a skillet over medium heat.
2. Add the ground beef and cook until browned.
3. Add zucchini slices, cooking until tender, and season with salt, pepper, and garlic powder.

NUTRITION FACTS:

- Calories: 420, Protein: 32g, Carbs: 6g, Fat: 32g

Dinner: Lemon Garlic Shrimp

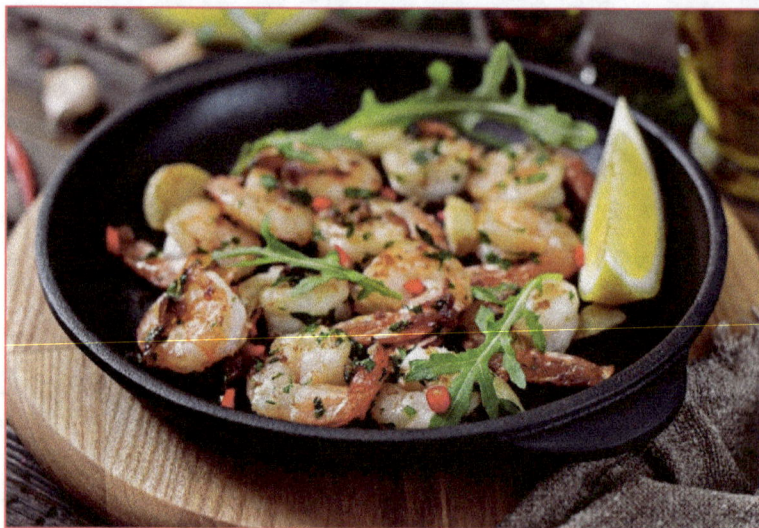

INGREDIENTS:

- 5 oz shrimp, peeled and deveined
- 1 tbsp olive oil
- 1 tbsp lemon juice
- Salt, pepper, and garlic powder to taste

INSTRUCTIONS:

1. Heat olive oil in a skillet over medium heat. Add shrimp to the skillet, season with salt, pepper, and garlic powder, and cook until pink and cooked through (about 4-5 minutes).
2. Drizzle with lemon juice just before serving.

TOTAL NUTRITION FOR DAY 6:

- Calories: 1040 Protein: 82g Carbs: 14g Fat: 76g

NUTRITION FACTS:

- Calories: 320, Protein: 35g, Carbs: 2g, Fat: 20g

Day 7 Reminder

Hydration & Reflection: Keep hydrated and take a few moments to reflect on the past week's progress.

Celebrate Small Wins: No matter how small, acknowledge your efforts. Each day brings you closer to your goals.

Today's Mantra: "I am stronger, healthier, and more resilient with each choice I make."

Breakfast: Steak & Eggs

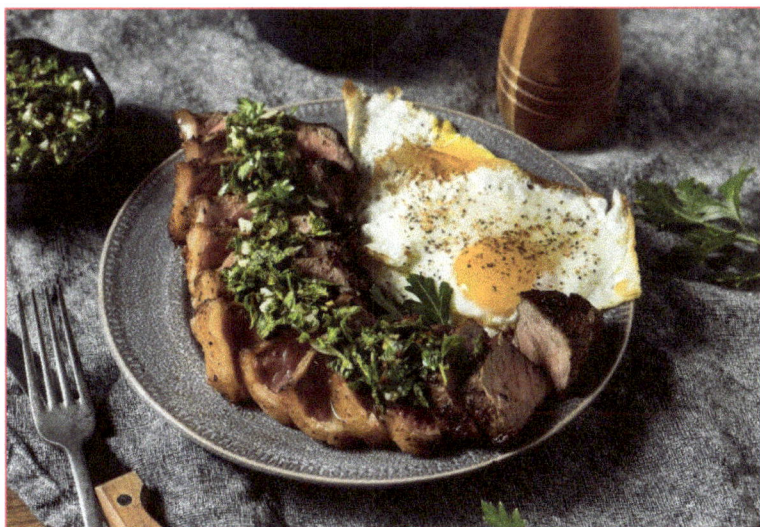

INGREDIENTS:

- 4 oz steak (any cut you prefer)
- 2 large eggs
- Salt and pepper to taste

INSTRUCTIONS:

1. Heat a skillet over medium-high heat and cook the steak to your desired doneness. Season with salt and pepper.
2. In a separate pan, cook the eggs to your liking (scrambled, fried, or poached). Serve the steak and eggs together.

NUTRITION FACTS:

- Calories: 450, Protein: 38g, Carbs: 1g, Fat: 34g

Lunch: Chicken Caesar Salad

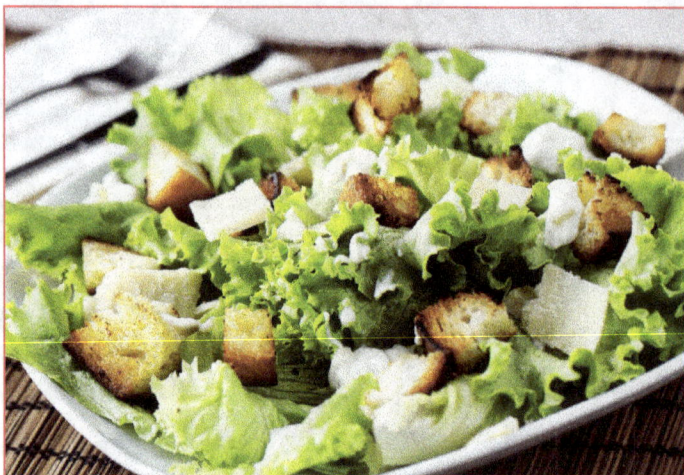

INGREDIENTS:

- 5 oz grilled chicken breast, sliced
- 2 cups romaine lettuce, chopped
- 1 tbsp Caesar dressing (no added sugar)
- Salt and pepper to taste

INSTRUCTIONS:

1. Arrange the chopped romaine on a plate and top with sliced grilled chicken.
2. Drizzle Caesar dressing over the salad, season with salt and pepper, and enjoy.

NUTRITION FACTS:

- Calories: 370, Protein: 32g, Carbs: 6g, Fat: 24g

Dinner: Baked Cod with Steamed Spinach

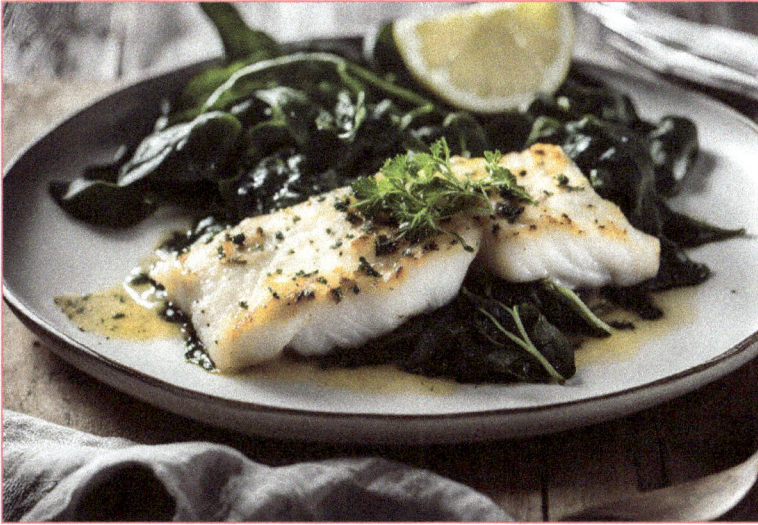

INGREDIENTS:

- 5 oz cod fillet
- 1 cup spinach
- 1 tbsp olive oil
- Salt, pepper, and garlic powder to taste

INSTRUCTIONS:

1. Preheat the oven to 375°F (190°C).
2. Place the cod on a baking sheet, drizzle with olive oil, and season with salt, pepper, and garlic powder. Bake for 12-15 minutes or until the fish flakes easily with a fork.

3. While the cod is baking, steam the spinach in a pot with a little water until wilted. Serve cod with the spinach.

TOTAL NUTRITION FOR DAY 7:

- Calories: 1140 Protein: 106g Carbs: 11g Fat: 76g

NUTRITION FACTS:

- Calories: 320, Protein: 36g, Carbs: 4g, Fat: 18g

Day 8 Reminder

Stay Hydrated & Rested: Remember to stay hydrated and prioritize rest today. Small steps lead to big results.

Focus on Consistency: Even on challenging days, staying consistent brings you closer to your goals.

Today's Mantra: "Each choice I make strengthens my commitment to my health."

Breakfast: Veggie Omelette with Spinach & Mushrooms

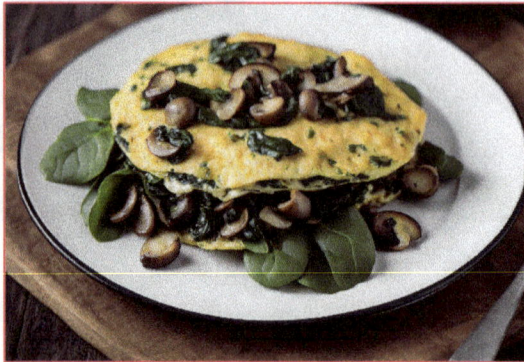

INGREDIENTS:

- 3 large eggs 1/2 cup spinach
- 1/4 cup mushrooms, sliced
- Salt and pepper to taste
- 1 tsp olive oil

INSTRUCTIONS:

1. Heat olive oil in a skillet over medium heat. Add mushrooms and spinach, cooking until softened.
2. In a bowl, whisk the eggs with salt and pepper, then pour over the veggies in the pan.
3. Let the eggs set and cook, folding gently for an even texture.

NUTRITION FACTS:

- Calories: 350, Protein: 21g, Carbs: 4g, Fat: 28g

Lunch: Shrimp & Avocado Salad

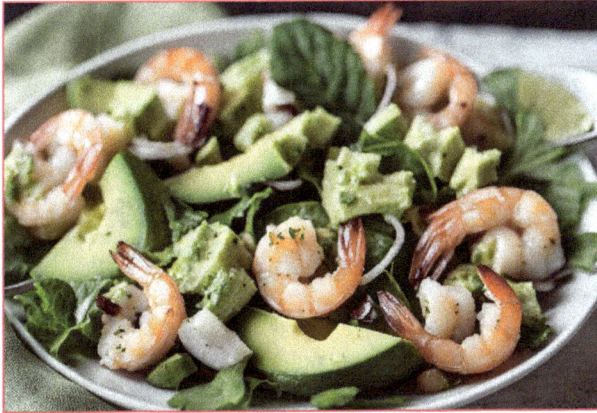

INGREDIENTS:

- 5 oz cooked shrimp
- 1/2 avocado, diced
- 2 cups mixed greens
- 1 tbsp olive oil
- Salt, pepper, and lemon juice to taste

INSTRUCTIONS:

1. Arrange mixed greens on a plate and top with cooked shrimp and avocado.
2. Drizzle with olive oil and a squeeze of lemon juice, then season with salt and pepper.

NUTRITION FACTS:

- Calories: 420, Protein: 30g, Carbs: 6g, Fat: 34g

Dinner: Grilled Salmon & Steamed Asparagus

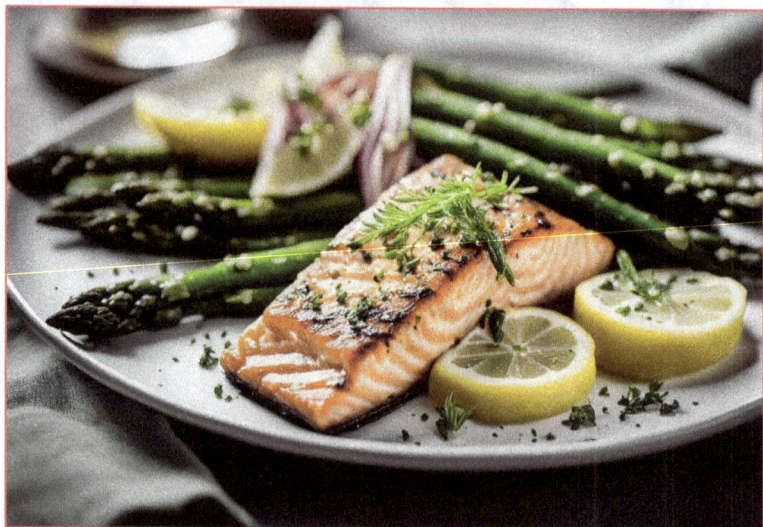

INGREDIENTS:

- 5 oz salmon filet
- 1 cup asparagus spears
- 1 tsp olive oil
- Salt, pepper, and lemon zest

INSTRUCTIONS:

1. Preheat the grill or a skillet to medium-high heat. Season the salmon with salt, pepper, and lemon zest.
2. Grill salmon for 4-5 minutes per side or until it flakes easily with a fork.

3. Steam asparagus in a pot with a small amount of water for 5-7 minutes until tender.

TOTAL NUTRITION FOR DAY 8:

- Calories: 1190 Protein: 89g Carbs: 14g Fat: 90g

NUTRITION FACTS:

- Calories: 420, Protein: 38g, Carbs: 4g, Fat: 28g

Day 9 Reminder

Mindfulness in Meals: Savor each bite, and take time to appreciate the nutritious foods you're eating.

Small Wins Matter: Celebrate each small victory, as they build the foundation for lasting change.

Today's Mantra: "I am worthy of the care I give myself."

Breakfast: Greek Yogurt with Berries (if dairy-tolerant)

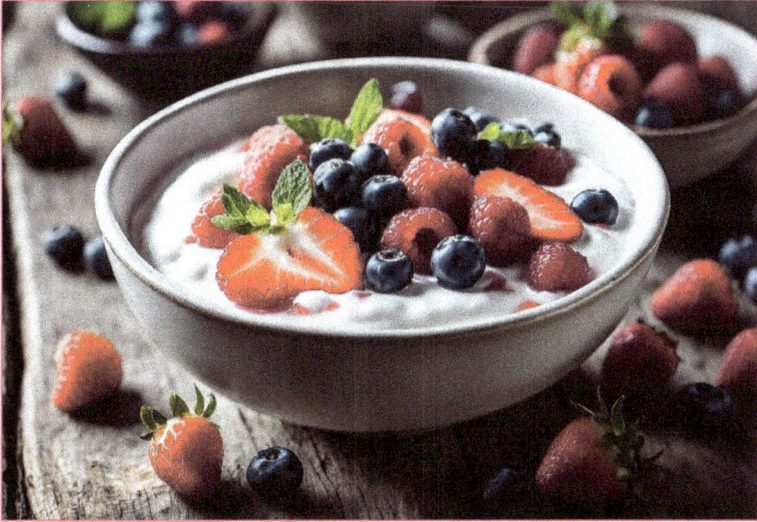

INGREDIENTS:

- 1/2 cup plain Greek yogurt (unsweetened)
- 1/4 cup mixed berries

INSTRUCTIONS:

1. Place Greek yogurt in a bowl and top with mixed berries.

NUTRITION FACTS:

- Calories: 180, Protein: 15g, Carbs: 10g, Fat: 8g

Lunch: Chicken & Bell Pepper Stir-Fry

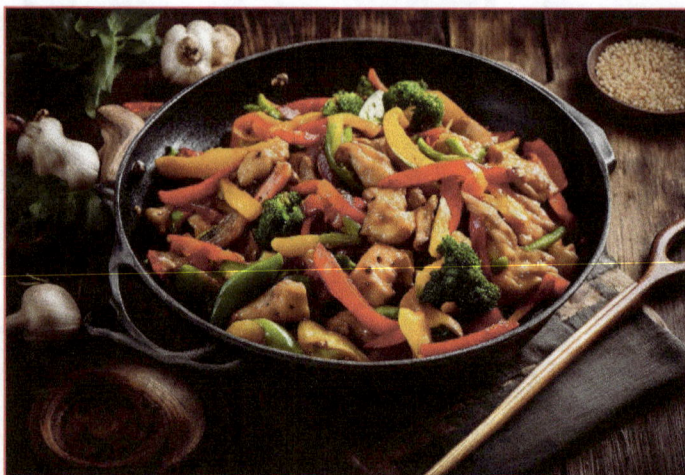

INGREDIENTS:

- 5 oz chicken breast, sliced
- 1/2 cup bell peppers, sliced
- 1 tbsp olive oil
- Salt, pepper, and garlic powder to taste

INSTRUCTIONS:

1. Heat olive oil in a skillet over medium heat. Add chicken slices and cook until golden brown, about 5 minutes.
2. Add bell pepper slices, cooking until tender. Season with salt, pepper, and garlic powder.

NUTRITION FACTS:

- Calories: 380, Protein: 35g, Carbs: 6g, Fat: 25g

Dinner: Tilapia with Green Beans

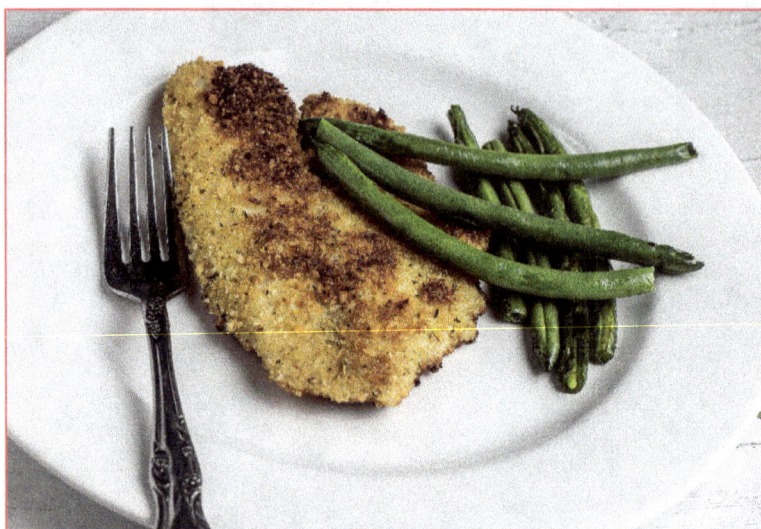

INGREDIENTS:

- 5 oz tilapia filet
- 1 cup green beans, steamed
- 1 tsp olive oil
- Salt and pepper to taste

INSTRUCTIONS:

1. Heat olive oil in a skillet over medium heat. Season the tilapia with salt and pepper.
2. Cook tilapia for 3-4 minutes per side or until it's flaky.
3. Steam green beans in a pot with a small amount of water until tender.

TOTAL NUTRITION FOR DAY 9:

- Calories: 850 Protein: 80g Carbs: 21g Fat: 48g

NUTRITION FACTS:

- Calories: 290, Protein: 30g, Carbs: 5g, Fat: 15g

Day 10 Reminder

Reflect on Your Journey: You've completed 10 days of focused eating. Reflect on the changes you've noticed and the progress you've made.

Keep the Momentum Going: Think about how you can carry these habits forward for lasting success.

Today's Mantra: "I am proud of my commitment to my health and well- being."

Breakfast: Scrambled Eggs with Turkey Sausage

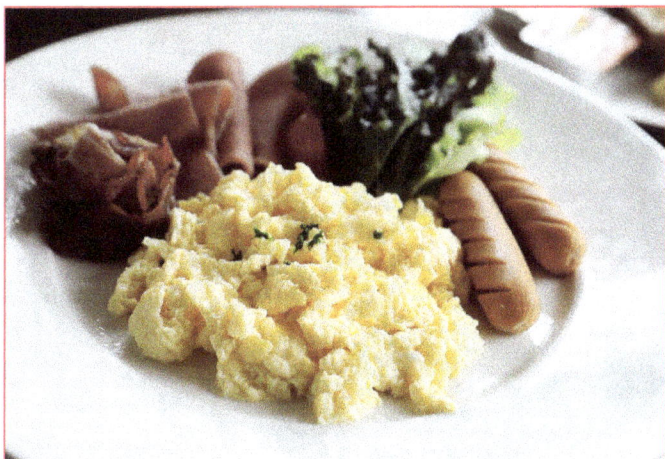

INGREDIENTS:

- 2 large eggs
- 2 oz turkey sausage (uncooked weight)
- Salt and pepper to taste

INSTRUCTIONS:

1. Cook turkey sausage in a skillet over medium heat until browned.
2. In the same skillet, scramble the eggs with salt and pepper until fully cooked.

NUTRITION FACTS:

- Calories: 320, Protein: 22g, Carbs: 2g, Fat: 24g

Lunch: Tuna Salad on Mixed Greens

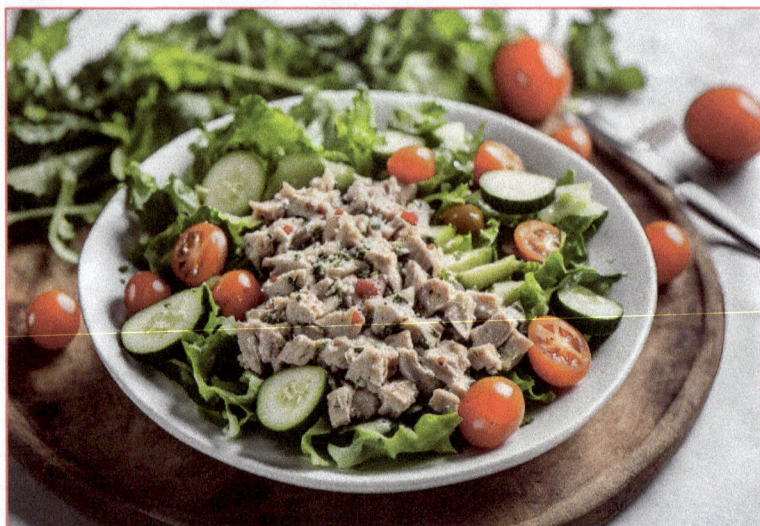

INGREDIENTS:

- 1 can tuna in water, drained (about 5 oz)
- 2 cups mixed greens
- 1 tbsp olive oil or mayonnaise
- Salt and pepper to taste

INSTRUCTIONS:

1. Mix tuna with olive oil or mayonnaise and season with salt and pepper.
2. Serve over mixed greens for a fresh, protein- packed salad.

NUTRITION FACTS:

- Calories: 300, Protein: 30g, Carbs: 3g, Fat: 18g

Dinner: Baked Chicken Thighs with Broccoli

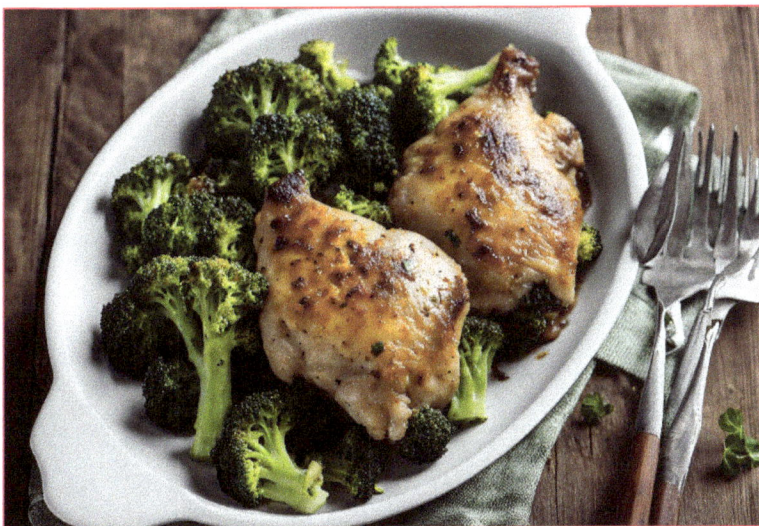

INGREDIENTS:

- 5 oz chicken thigh
- 1 cup broccoli, steamed
- Salt, pepper, and garlic powder to taste

INSTRUCTIONS:

1. Preheat the oven to 375°F (190°C). Season chicken thighs with salt, pepper, and garlic powder.
2. Bake chicken for 25-30 minutes or until fully cooked.
3. Steam broccoli in a pot until tender.

TOTAL NUTRITION FOR DAY 10:

- Calories: 1040 Protein: 82g Carbs: 9g Fat: 72g

NUTRITION FACTS:

- Calories: 420, Protein: 30g, Carbs: 4g, Fat: 30g

DAILY PLANNER

Day   1

Today, I Will Focus On

_____

_____

_____

🧺 Meal Tracker

🍞 Breakfast _____

Changes/Addition: _____

🛎 Lunch _____

Changes/Addition: _____

🍜 Dinner _____

Changes/Addition: _____

Water Intake 🥤 🥤 🥤 🥤 🥤 🥤 🥤 🥤 🥤 🥤

💪 Workout Log
Workout Type (Circle One)

○ Strength Training   ○ Cardio   ○ Flexibility

Workout Details (e.g., Upper Body, Lower Body, Running, etc.) _____

Duration	Intensity	Achievements/Adjustments

What went well today? _____

What challenges did I face? _____

How did I feel overall? _____

DAILY JOURNAL

Day

Today's Thoughts and Reflections

_____

_____

_____

_____

_____

_____

_____

_____

_____

_____

_____

_____

Gratitude

_____

_____

_____

_____

_____

DAILY PLANNER

Day   2

Today, I Will Focus On

_____

_____

_____

🧺 Meal Tracker

🍞 Breakfast _____

Changes/Addition: _____

🛎 Lunch _____

Changes/Addition: _____

🍲 Dinner _____

Changes/Addition: _____

Water Intake 🥤 🥤 🥤 🥤 🥤 🥤 🥤 🥤 🥤 🥤

💪 Workout Log
Workout Type (Circle One)

○   Strength Training   ○ Cardio   ○ Flexibility

Workout Details (e.g., Upper Body, Lower Body, Running, etc.) _____

Duration	Intensity	Achievements/Adjustments

What went well today? _____

What challenges did I face? _____

How did I feel overall? _____

DAILY JOURNAL

Day

Today's Thoughts and Reflections

_____

_____

_____

_____

_____

_____

_____

_____

_____

_____

_____

_____

_____

Gratitude

_____

_____

_____

_____

_____

DAILY PLANNER

Day   3

Today, I Will Focus On

_____

_____

_____

🧺 Meal Tracker

🍞 Breakfast _____

Changes/Addition: _____

🔔 Lunch _____

Changes/Addition: _____

🍜 Dinner _____

Changes/Addition: _____

Water Intake   🥛   🥛   🥛   🥛   🥛   🥛   🥛   🥛   🥛   🥛

💪 Workout Log
Workout Type (Circle One)

○   Strength Training   ○ Cardio   ○   Flexibility

Workout Details (e.g., Upper Body, Lower Body, Running, etc.) _____

Duration	Intensity	Achievements/Adjustments

What went well today? _____

What challenges did I face? _____

How did I feel overall? _____

DAILY JOURNAL

Day

Today's Thoughts and Reflections

_____

_____

_____

_____

_____

_____

_____

_____

_____

_____

_____

_____

Gratitude

_____

_____

_____

_____

_____

DAILY PLANNER

Day   4

Today, I Will Focus On

_____

_____

_____

🧺 Meal Tracker

🍞 Breakfast _____

Changes/Addition: _____

🔔 Lunch _____

Changes/Addition: _____

🍜 Dinner _____

Changes/Addition: _____

Water Intake   🥤 🥤 🥤 🥤 🥤 🥤 🥤 🥤 🥤 🥤

💪 Workout Log
Workout Type (Circle One)

○   Strength Training   ○ Cardio   ○   Flexibility

Workout Details (e.g., Upper Body, Lower Body, Running, etc.) _____

Duration	Intensity	Achievements/Adjustments

What went well today? _____

What challenges did I face? _____

How did I feel overall? _____

DAILY JOURNAL

Day

Today's Thoughts and Reflections

_____

_____

_____

_____

_____

_____

_____

_____

_____

_____

_____

_____

_____

_____

_____

Gratitude

_____

_____

_____

_____

_____

_____

DAILY PLANNER

Day   5

Today, I Will Focus On

_____

_____

_____

🧺 Meal Tracker

🍞 Breakfast _____

Changes/Addition: _____

🔔 Lunch _____

Changes/Addition: _____

🍲 Dinner _____

Changes/Addition: _____

Water Intake 🥛 🥛 🥛 🥛 🥛 🥛 🥛 🥛 🥛 🥛

💪 Workout Log
Workout Type (Circle One)

○ Strength Training   ○ Cardio   ○ Flexibility

Workout Details (e.g., Upper Body, Lower Body, Running, etc.) _____

Duration	Intensity	Achievements/Adjustments

What went well today? _____

What challenges did I face? _____

How did I feel overall? _____

DAILY JOURNAL

Day

Today's Thoughts and Reflections

_____

_____

_____

_____

_____

_____

_____

_____

_____

_____

_____

_____

Gratitude

_____

_____

_____

_____

_____

DAILY PLANNER

Day   6

Today, I Will Focus On

_____

_____

_____

🧺 Meal Tracker

🍞 Breakfast _____

Changes/Addition: _____

🛎 Lunch _____

Changes/Addition: _____

🍲 Dinner _____

Changes/Addition: _____

Water Intake   🥛 🥛 🥛 🥛 🥛 🥛 🥛 🥛 🥛 🥛

💪 Workout Log
Workout Type (Circle One)

○   Strength Training   ○ Cardio   ○   Flexibility

Workout Details (e.g., Upper Body, Lower Body, Running, etc.) _____

Duration	Intensity	Achievements/Adjustments

What went well today? _____

What challenges did I face? _____

How did I feel overall? _____

DAILY JOURNAL

Day

Today's Thoughts and Reflections

_____
_____
_____
_____
_____
_____
_____
_____
_____
_____
_____
_____

Gratitude

_____
_____
_____
_____
_____
_____

DAILY PLANNER

Day   7

Today, I Will Focus On

_____

_____

_____

🧺 Meal Tracker

🍞 Breakfast _____

Changes/Addition: _____

🛎 Lunch _____

Changes/Addition: _____

🍲 Dinner _____

Changes/Addition: _____

Water Intake   🥛 🥛 🥛 🥛 🥛 🥛 🥛 🥛 🥛 🥛

💪 Workout Log
Workout Type (Circle One)

○ Strength Training   ○ Cardio   ○ Flexibility

Workout Details (e.g., Upper Body, Lower Body, Running, etc.) _____

Duration	Intensity	Achievements/Adjustments

What went well today? _____

What challenges did I face? _____

How did I feel overall? _____

DAILY JOURNAL

Day

Today's Thoughts and Reflections

_____

_____

_____

_____

_____

_____

_____

_____

_____

_____

_____

_____

_____

Gratitude

_____

_____

_____

_____

_____

DAILY PLANNER

Day   8

Today, I Will Focus On

_____

_____

_____

🧺 Meal Tracker

🍞 Breakfast _____

Changes/Addition: _____

🔔 Lunch _____

Changes/Addition: _____

🍲 Dinner _____

Changes/Addition: _____

Water Intake 🥛 🥛 🥛 🥛 🥛 🥛 🥛 🥛 🥛 🥛

💪 Workout Log
Workout Type (Circle One)

○   Strength Training   ○ Cardio   ○ Flexibility

Workout Details (e.g., Upper Body, Lower Body, Running, etc.) _____

Duration	Intensity	Achievements/Adjustments

What went well today? _____

What challenges did I face? _____

How did I feel overall? _____

DAILY JOURNAL

Day

Today's Thoughts and Reflections

_____
_____
_____
_____
_____
_____
_____
_____
_____
_____
_____
_____
_____

Gratitude

_____
_____
_____
_____
_____

DAILY PLANNER

Day   9

Today, I Will Focus On

_____

_____

_____

🧺 Meal Tracker

🍞 Breakfast _____

Changes/Addition: _____

🔔 Lunch _____

Changes/Addition: _____

🍲 Dinner _____

Changes/Addition: _____

Water Intake   🥛 🥛 🥛 🥛 🥛 🥛 🥛 🥛 🥛 🥛

💪 Workout Log
Workout Type (Circle One)

○ Strength Training   ○ Cardio   ○ Flexibility

Workout Details (e.g., Upper Body, Lower Body, Running, etc.) _____

Duration	Intensity	Achievements/Adjustments

What went well today? _____

What challenges did I face? _____

How did I feel overall? _____

DAILY JOURNAL

Day

Today's Thoughts and Reflections

_____

_____

_____

_____

_____

_____

_____

_____

_____

_____

_____

_____

_____

Gratitude

_____

_____

_____

_____

_____

_____

DAILY PLANNER

Day   10

Today, I Will Focus On

_____

_____

_____

🧺 Meal Tracker

🍞 Breakfast _____

Changes/Addition: _____

🔔 Lunch _____

Changes/Addition: _____

🍲 Dinner _____

Changes/Addition: _____

Water Intake   🥛 🥛 🥛 🥛 🥛 🥛 🥛 🥛 🥛 🥛

💪 Workout Log
Workout Type (Circle One)

○ Strength Training   ○ Cardio   ○ Flexibility

Workout Details (e.g., Upper Body, Lower Body, Running, etc.) _____

Duration	Intensity	Achievements/Adjustments

What went well today? _____

What challenges did I face? _____

How did I feel overall? _____

DAILY JOURNAL

Day

Today's Thoughts and Reflections

_____

_____

_____

_____

_____

_____

_____

_____

_____

_____

_____

_____

_____

_____

Gratitude

_____

_____

_____

_____

_____

_____

CONGRATULATIONS ON COMPLETING THE 10-DAY RAPID WEIGHT LOSS PLAN!

You did it! Reaching the end of these 10 days is a huge accomplishment, and I hope you take a moment to truly celebrate yourself for the commitment and effort you've put in. This wasn't just about following a meal and exercise plan it was about prioritizing your health, making intentional choices, and starting the process of becoming the best version of yourself. I'm so proud of you for showing up for yourself.

But let me be clear: this is not the end—it's just the beginning.

These 10 days were designed to give you a jumpstart, to show you what's possible when you align your meals, movement, and mindset. You now have a solid foundation, and you can choose where to go from here.

You have a few options moving forward, and every one of them is valid:

- You can repeat this 10-day plan as many times as you need to. Consistency is powerful, and going through these 10 days again can help reinforce the habits you're building.
- You can use the approved foods list to create your own meals. This gives you flexibility and variety while sticking to the principles you've learned about balanced eating.
- Or, if you're ready to dive deeper, you can take the next step with my Menopause Weight Loss Blueprint.

What's Next?

About the Menopause Weight Loss Blueprint

If you're looking for a more comprehensive, done-for-you program, the Menopause Weight Loss Blueprint is designed to take you even further. It's not just a weight-loss plan—it's a complete guide to navigating menopause with confidence, clarity, and control.

Here's what you'll find inside:

- Intermittent Fasting Strategies: Learn how to incorporate fasting into your lifestyle in a way that works with your hormones and supports sustainable weight loss.
- Deeper Nutritional Guidance: Discover how to further optimize your eating habits to support bone density, hormonal health, and metabolism.
- BHRT Education: Get a deeper dive into bioidentical hormone replacement therapy (BHRT)—what it is, how it works, and whether it's the right choice for you.
- Bone Density Support: Explore exercises and supplements that help protect your bones as you age, keeping you strong and resilient.
- Mindset and Emotional Wellness: Learn how to address emotional triggers, build a resilient mindset, and stay consistent even when life throws you a curveball.
- Customizable Meal Plans and Recipes: More recipes, meal planning tools, and strategies to help you stay on track while enjoying the foods you love.
- Accountability Tools: More tracking sheets, journaling prompts, and tips to keep you focused on your goals.

The Blueprint is all about making the menopause journey easier, more manageable, and tailored to YOU. It's like having me as your personal coach, guiding you step by step.

Continuing Your Journey

No matter which path you choose, I've included extra tracker and journal pages at the end of this book to support you. Whether you're repeating this plan for another 10 days, extending it to 20 or 30 days, or transitioning to your own meal plan, you'll have the tools to stay on track. Use these pages to keep logging your meals, tracking your weight, and reflecting on your progress.

Remember, this is YOUR journey, and there's no one-size-fits-all timeline. Whether you reach your goals in 10 days, 30 days, or beyond, the most important thing is that you keep showing up for yourself.

A FINAL THOUGHT

You've already taken such an incredible step by starting this journey. Change isn't easy, but you're doing it. You've committed to your health, well-being, and future, which is something to be proud of. Every small choice you make builds momentum. Every meal, every workout, every reflection gets you closer to the person you want to be.

I'm honored to have been part of your journey, and I'd love to see where it takes you. You can email me at menopause@michelleabates.com and let me know about your results. Keep believing in yourself, keep making progress, and know that you are capable of so much more than you think.

Congratulations again—you've got this! With love and encouragement,

Coach Michelle A Bates, INHC

Not Ending Your Journey Just Yet

For Those Continuing on Your Journey

As a bonus to help you stay on track, I've included 21 days of additional tracker pages—just like the ones you used during your first 10 days. Use these pages to record your meals, exercise, weight, and reflections for as many days as you need—whether it's another 10 days, 21 days, or even longer.

This is your journey, and you're in full control. The tools are here to support you every step of the way. Remember, every day is another opportunity to prioritize your health, listen to your body, and make choices that align with your goals.

You've already taken an incredible step, and I know you'll continue to do amazing things. Keep going—you've got this!

DAILY PLANNER

Day _____

Today, I Will Focus On

_____

_____

_____

🧺 Meal Tracker

🍞 Breakfast _____

Changes/Addition: _____

🔔 Lunch _____

Changes/Addition: _____

🍲 Dinner _____

Changes/Addition: _____

Water Intake 🥛 🥛 🥛 🥛 🥛 🥛 🥛 🥛 🥛 🥛

💪 Workout Log

Workout Type (Circle One)

○ Strength Training   ○ Cardio   ○ Flexibility

Workout Details (e.g., Upper Body, Lower Body, Running, etc.) _____

Duration	Intensity	Achievements/Adjustments

What went well today? _____

What challenges did I face? _____

How did I feel overall? _____

DAILY JOURNAL

Day

Today's Thoughts and Reflections

_____
_____
_____
_____
_____
_____
_____
_____
_____
_____
_____
_____

Gratitude

_____
_____
_____
_____
_____
_____

DAILY PLANNER

Day _____

Today, I Will Focus On

_____

_____

_____

🧺 Meal Tracker

🍞 Breakfast _____

Changes/Addition: _____

🔔 Lunch _____

Changes/Addition: _____

🍲 Dinner _____

Changes/Addition: _____

Water Intake 🥛 🥛 🥛 🥛 🥛 🥛 🥛 🥛 🥛 🥛

💪 Workout Log

Workout Type (Circle One)

○ Strength Training   ○ Cardio   ○ Flexibility

Workout Details (e.g., Upper Body, Lower Body, Running, etc.) _____

Duration	Intensity	Achievements/Adjustments

What went well today? _____

What challenges did I face? _____

How did I feel overall? _____

DAILY JOURNAL

Day

Today's Thoughts and Reflections

_____
_____
_____
_____
_____
_____
_____
_____
_____
_____
_____
_____
_____

Gratitude

_____
_____
_____
_____
_____
_____

DAILY PLANNER

Day _____

Today, I Will Focus On

_____

_____

_____

🧺 Meal Tracker

🍞 Breakfast _____

Changes/Addition: _____

🔔 Lunch _____

Changes/Addition: _____

🍲 Dinner _____

Changes/Addition: _____

Water Intake 🥛 🥛 🥛 🥛 🥛 🥛 🥛 🥛 🥛 🥛

💪 Workout Log

Workout Type (Circle One)

○ Strength Training   ○ Cardio   ○ Flexibility

Workout Details (e.g., Upper Body, Lower Body, Running, etc.) _____

Duration	Intensity	Achievements/Adjustments

What went well today? _____

What challenges did I face? _____

How did I feel overall? _____

DAILY JOURNAL

Day

Today's Thoughts and Reflections

_____
_____
_____
_____
_____
_____
_____
_____
_____
_____
_____
_____
_____
_____

Gratitude

_____
_____
_____
_____
_____
_____

DAILY PLANNER

Day _____

Today, I Will Focus On

_____

_____

_____

🧺 Meal Tracker

🍞 Breakfast _____

Changes/Addition: _____

🔔 Lunch _____

Changes/Addition: _____

🍲 Dinner _____

Changes/Addition: _____

Water Intake 🥤 🥤 🥤 🥤 🥤 🥤 🥤 🥤 🥤 🥤

💪 Workout Log

Workout Type (Circle One)

○ Strength Training   ○ Cardio   ○ Flexibility

Workout Details (e.g., Upper Body, Lower Body, Running, etc.)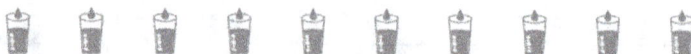

Duration	Intensity	Achievements/Adjustments

What went well today? _____

What challenges did I face? _____

How did I feel overall? _____

DAILY JOURNAL

Day

Today's Thoughts and Reflections

_____

_____

_____

_____

_____

_____

_____

_____

_____

_____

_____

_____

_____

Gratitude

_____

_____

_____

_____

_____

DAILY PLANNER

Day _____

Today, I Will Focus On

_____

_____

_____

🧺 Meal Tracker

🍞 Breakfast _____

Changes/Addition: _____

🛎 Lunch _____

Changes/Addition: _____

🍲 Dinner _____

Changes/Addition: _____

Water Intake   🥤 🥤 🥤 🥤 🥤 🥤 🥤 🥤 🥤 🥤

💪 Workout Log

Workout Type (Circle One)

○ Strength Training   ○ Cardio   ○ Flexibility

Workout Details (e.g., Upper Body, Lower Body, Running, etc.) _____

Duration	Intensity	Achievements/Adjustments

What went well today? _____

What challenges did I face? _____

How did I feel overall? _____

DAILY JOURNAL

Day

Today's Thoughts and Reflections

_____

_____

_____

_____

_____

_____

_____

_____

_____

_____

_____

_____

_____

_____

Gratitude

_____

_____

_____

_____

_____

_____

DAILY PLANNER

Day

Today, I Will Focus On

_____

_____

_____

🧺 Meal Tracker

🍞 Breakfast _____

Changes/Addition: _____

🔔 Lunch _____

Changes/Addition: _____

🍲 Dinner _____

Changes/Addition: _____

Water Intake 🥛 🥛 🥛 🥛 🥛 🥛 🥛 🥛 🥛 🥛

🎯 Workout Log

Workout Type (Circle One)

○ Strength Training   ○ Cardio   ○ Flexibility

Workout Details (e.g., Upper Body, Lower Body, Running, etc.)

Duration	Intensity	Achievements/Adjustments

What went well today? _____

What challenges did I face? _____

How did I feel overall? _____

DAILY JOURNAL

Day

Today's Thoughts and Reflections

_____

_____

_____

_____

_____

_____

_____

_____

_____

_____

_____

_____

_____

Gratitude

_____

_____

_____

_____

_____

DAILY PLANNER

Day

Today, I Will Focus On

_____

_____

_____

🧺 Meal Tracker

🍞 Breakfast _____

Changes/Addition: _____

🔔 Lunch _____

Changes/Addition: _____

🍲 Dinner _____

Changes/Addition: _____

Water Intake 🥤 🥤 🥤 🥤 🥤 🥤 🥤 🥤 🥤 🥤

🏋️ Workout Log

Workout Type (Circle One)

○ Strength Training   ○ Cardio   ○ Flexibility

Workout Details (e.g., Upper Body, Lower Body, Running, etc.) _____

Duration	Intensity	Achievements/Adjustments

What went well today? _____

What challenges did I face? _____

How did I feel overall? _____

DAILY JOURNAL

Day

Today's Thoughts and Reflections

_____

_____

_____

_____

_____

_____

_____

_____

_____

_____

_____

_____

_____

Gratitude

_____

_____

_____

_____

_____

DAILY PLANNER

Day

Today, I Will Focus On

_____

_____

_____

🧺 Meal Tracker

🍞 Breakfast _____

Changes/Addition: _____

🔔 Lunch _____

Changes/Addition: _____

🍲 Dinner _____

Changes/Addition: _____

Water Intake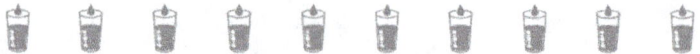

💪 Workout Log

Workout Type (Circle One)

○ Strength Training   ○ Cardio   ○ Flexibility

Workout Details (e.g., Upper Body, Lower Body, Running, etc.) _____

Duration	Intensity	Achievements/Adjustments

What went well today? _____

What challenges did I face? _____

How did I feel overall? _____

DAILY JOURNAL

Day

Today's Thoughts and Reflections

_____
_____
_____
_____
_____
_____
_____
_____
_____
_____
_____
_____
_____
_____

Gratitude

_____
_____
_____
_____
_____
_____

DAILY PLANNER

Day

Today, I Will Focus On

_____

_____

_____

🧺 Meal Tracker

🍞 Breakfast _____

Changes/Addition: _____

🔔 Lunch _____

Changes/Addition: _____

🍲 Dinner _____

Changes/Addition: _____

Water Intake 🥤 🥤 🥤 🥤 🥤 🥤 🥤 🥤 🥤 🥤

🏋️ Workout Log

Workout Type (Circle One)

○ Strength Training   ○ Cardio   ○ Flexibility

Workout Details (e.g., Upper Body, Lower Body, Running, etc.)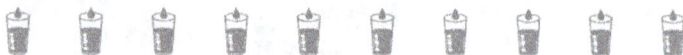

Duration	Intensity	Achievements/Adjustments

What went well today? _____

What challenges did I face? _____

How did I feel overall? _____

DAILY JOURNAL

Day

Today's Thoughts and Reflections

_____

_____

_____

_____

_____

_____

_____

_____

_____

_____

_____

_____

_____

_____

Gratitude

_____

_____

_____

_____

_____

_____

DAILY PLANNER

Day _____

Today, I Will Focus On

_____

_____

_____

🍞 Meal Tracker

🍞 Breakfast _____

Changes/Addition: _____

🔔 Lunch _____

Changes/Addition: _____

🍲 Dinner _____

Changes/Addition: _____

Water Intake   🥤 🥤 🥤 🥤 🥤 🥤 🥤 🥤 🥤 🥤

💪 Workout Log

Workout Type (Circle One)

○ Strength Training   ○ Cardio   ○ Flexibility

Workout Details (e.g., Upper Body, Lower Body, Running, etc.) _____

Duration	Intensity	Achievements/Adjustments

What went well today? _____

What challenges did I face? _____

How did I feel overall? _____

DAILY JOURNAL

Day

Today's Thoughts and Reflections

_____
_____
_____
_____
_____
_____
_____
_____
_____
_____
_____
_____
_____
_____
_____

Gratitude

_____
_____
_____
_____
_____

DAILY PLANNER

Day

Today, I Will Focus On

_____

_____

_____

🧺 Meal Tracker

🍞 Breakfast _____

Changes/Addition: _____

🔔 Lunch _____

Changes/Addition: _____

🍲 Dinner _____

Changes/Addition: _____

Water Intake 🥛 🥛 🥛 🥛 🥛 🥛 🥛 🥛 🥛 🥛

💪 Workout Log

Workout Type (Circle One)

○   Strength Training   ○ Cardio   ○ Flexibility

Workout Details (e.g., Upper Body, Lower Body, Running, etc.) _____

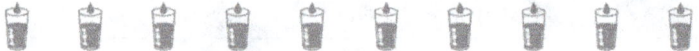

Duration	Intensity	Achievements/Adjustments

What went well today? _____

What challenges did I face? _____

How did I feel overall? _____

DAILY JOURNAL

Day

Today's Thoughts and Reflections

_____
_____
_____
_____
_____
_____
_____
_____
_____
_____
_____
_____
_____

Gratitude

_____
_____
_____
_____
_____
_____

DAILY PLANNER

Day

Today, I Will Focus On

_____

_____

_____

🧺 Meal Tracker

🍞 Breakfast _____

Changes/Addition: _____

🔔 Lunch _____

Changes/Addition: _____

🍲 Dinner _____

Changes/Addition: _____

Water Intake 🥤 🥤 🥤 🥤 🥤 🥤 🥤 🥤 🥤 🥤

💪 Workout Log
Workout Type (Circle One)

○ Strength Training   ○ Cardio   ○ Flexibility

Workout Details (e.g., Upper Body, Lower Body, Running, etc.)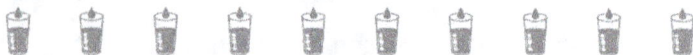

Duration	Intensity	Achievements/Adjustments

What went well today? _____

What challenges did I face? _____

How did I feel overall? _____

DAILY JOURNAL

Day

Today's Thoughts and Reflections

_____

_____

_____

_____

_____

_____

_____

_____

_____

_____

_____

_____

_____

Gratitude

_____

_____

_____

_____

_____

_____

DAILY PLANNER

Day _____

Today, I Will Focus On

_____

_____

_____

🧺 Meal Tracker

🍞 Breakfast _____

Changes/Addition: _____

🔔 Lunch _____

Changes/Addition: _____

🍲 Dinner _____

Changes/Addition: _____

Water Intake 🥤 🥤 🥤 🥤 🥤 🥤 🥤 🥤 🥤 🥤

💪 Workout Log

Workout Type (Circle One)

○ Strength Training   ○ Cardio   ○ Flexibility

Workout Details (e.g., Upper Body, Lower Body, Running, etc.) _____

Duration	Intensity	Achievements/Adjustments

What went well today? _____

What challenges did I face? _____

How did I feel overall? _____

DAILY JOURNAL

Day

Today's Thoughts and Reflections

_____

_____

_____

_____

_____

_____

_____

_____

_____

_____

_____

_____

_____

_____

Gratitude

_____

_____

_____

_____

_____

_____

DAILY PLANNER

Day _____

Today, I Will Focus On

_____

_____

_____

🧺 Meal Tracker

🍞 Breakfast _____

Changes/Addition: _____

🔔 Lunch _____

Changes/Addition: _____

🍲 Dinner _____

Changes/Addition: _____

Water Intake 🥛 🥛 🥛 🥛 🥛 🥛 🥛 🥛 🥛 🥛

💪 Workout Log

Workout Type (Circle One)

○ Strength Training   ○ Cardio   ○ Flexibility

Workout Details (e.g., Upper Body, Lower Body, Running, etc.) _____

Duration	Intensity	Achievements/Adjustments

What went well today? _____

What challenges did I face? _____

How did I feel overall? _____

DAILY JOURNAL

Day

Today's Thoughts and Reflections

_____
_____
_____
_____
_____
_____
_____
_____
_____
_____
_____
_____
_____

Gratitude

_____
_____
_____
_____
_____

DAILY PLANNER

Day _____

Today, I Will Focus On

_____

_____

_____

🧺 Meal Tracker

🍞 Breakfast _____

Changes/Addition: _____

🔔 Lunch _____

Changes/Addition: _____

🍲 Dinner _____

Changes/Addition: _____

Water Intake 🥤 🥤 🥤 🥤 🥤 🥤 🥤 🥤 🥤 🥤

💪 Workout Log

Workout Type (Circle One)

○ Strength Training   ○ Cardio   ○ Flexibility

Workout Details (e.g., Upper Body, Lower Body, Running, etc.) _____

Duration	Intensity	Achievements/Adjustments

What went well today? _____

What challenges did I face? _____

How did I feel overall? _____

DAILY JOURNAL

Day

Today's Thoughts and Reflections

_____
_____
_____
_____
_____
_____
_____
_____
_____
_____
_____
_____
_____
_____

Gratitude

_____
_____
_____
_____
_____
_____

DAILY PLANNER

Day _____

Today, I Will Focus On

_____

_____

_____

🍞 Meal Tracker

🍞 Breakfast _____

Changes/Addition: _____

🔔 Lunch _____

Changes/Addition: _____

🍲 Dinner _____

Changes/Addition: _____

Water Intake 🥛 🥛 🥛 🥛 🥛 🥛 🥛 🥛 🥛 🥛

💪 Workout Log

Workout Type (Circle One)

○ Strength Training   ○ Cardio   ○ Flexibility

Workout Details (e.g., Upper Body, Lower Body, Running, etc.) _____

Duration	Intensity	Achievements/Adjustments

What went well today? _____

What challenges did I face? _____

How did I feel overall? _____

DAILY JOURNAL

Day

Today's Thoughts and Reflections

_____
_____
_____
_____
_____
_____
_____
_____
_____
_____
_____
_____
_____
_____

Gratitude

_____
_____
_____
_____
_____
_____

DAILY PLANNER

Day �_____

Today, I Will Focus On

_____

_____

_____

🧺 Meal Tracker

🍞 Breakfast _____

Changes/Addition: _____

🔔 Lunch _____

Changes/Addition: _____

🍲 Dinner _____

Changes/Addition: _____

Water Intake 🥤 🥤 🥤 🥤 🥤 🥤 🥤 🥤 🥤 🥤

💪 Workout Log

Workout Type (Circle One)

○ Strength Training   ○ Cardio   ○ Flexibility

Workout Details (e.g., Upper Body, Lower Body, Running, etc.) _____

Duration	Intensity	Achievements/Adjustments

What went well today? _____

What challenges did I face? _____

How did I feel overall? _____

DAILY JOURNAL

Day

Today's Thoughts and Reflections

_____

_____

_____

_____

_____

_____

_____

_____

_____

_____

_____

_____

Gratitude

_____

_____

_____

_____

_____

_____

DAILY PLANNER

Day _____

Today, I Will Focus On

_____

_____

_____

🧺 Meal Tracker

🍞 Breakfast _____

Changes/Addition: _____

🔔 Lunch _____

Changes/Addition: _____

🍲 Dinner _____

Changes/Addition: _____

Water Intake 🥛 🥛 🥛 🥛 🥛 🥛 🥛 🥛 🥛 🥛

💪 Workout Log
Workout Type (Circle One)

○ Strength Training   ○ Cardio   ○ Flexibility

Workout Details (e.g., Upper Body, Lower Body, Running, etc.) _____

Duration	Intensity	Achievements/Adjustments

What went well today? _____

What challenges did I face? _____

How did I feel overall? _____

DAILY JOURNAL

Day

Today's Thoughts and Reflections

_____

_____

_____

_____

_____

_____

_____

_____

_____

_____

_____

Gratitude

_____

_____

_____

_____

_____

DAILY PLANNER

Day _____

Today, I Will Focus On

_____

_____

_____

🧺 Meal Tracker

🍞 Breakfast _____

Changes/Addition: _____

🔔 Lunch _____

Changes/Addition: _____

🍲 Dinner _____

Changes/Addition: _____

Water Intake 🥤 🥤 🥤 🥤 🥤 🥤 🥤 🥤 🥤 🥤

🎯 Workout Log

Workout Type (Circle One)

○ Strength Training   ○ Cardio   ○ Flexibility

Workout Details (e.g., Upper Body, Lower Body, Running, etc.) _____

Duration	Intensity	Achievements/Adjustments

What went well today? _____

What challenges did I face? _____

How did I feel overall? _____

DAILY JOURNAL

Day

Today's Thoughts and Reflections

_____
_____
_____
_____
_____
_____
_____
_____
_____
_____
_____
_____
_____
_____

Gratitude

_____
_____
_____
_____
_____
_____

DAILY PLANNER

Day _____

Today, I Will Focus On

_____

_____

_____

🧺 Meal Tracker

🍞 Breakfast _____

Changes/Addition: _____

🔔 Lunch _____

Changes/Addition: _____

🍲 Dinner _____

Changes/Addition: _____

Water Intake 🥤 🥤 🥤 🥤 🥤 🥤 🥤 🥤 🥤 🥤

💪 Workout Log

Workout Type (Circle One)

○ Strength Training　　　○ Cardio　　　○ Flexibility

Workout Details (e.g., Upper Body, Lower Body, Running, etc.) _____

Duration	Intensity	Achievements/Adjustments

What went well today? _____

What challenges did I face? _____

How did I feel overall? _____

DAILY JOURNAL

Day

Today's Thoughts and Reflections

_____

_____

_____

_____

_____

_____

_____

_____

_____

_____

_____

_____

_____

Gratitude

_____

_____

_____

_____

_____

_____

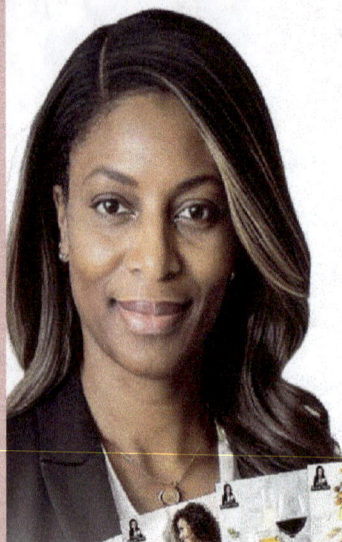

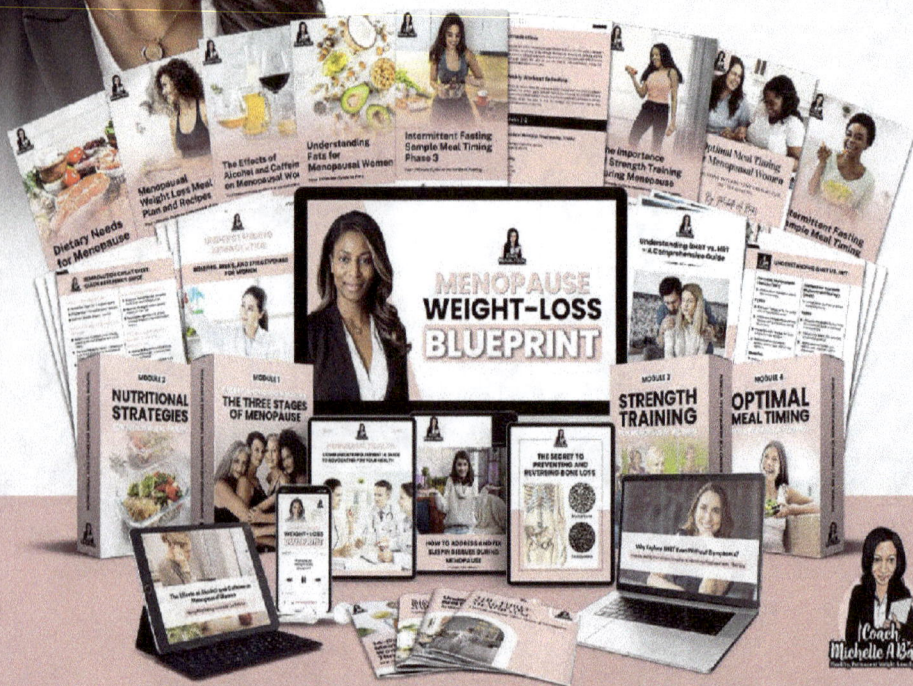

www.ingramcontent.com/pod-product-compliance
Lightning Source LLC
Chambersburg PA
CBHW070805270326
41927CB00010B/2295